Kicking Cancer in the Kitchen

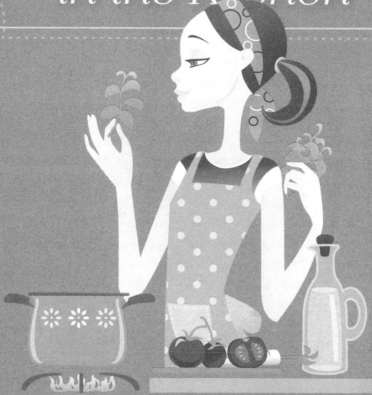

The Girlfriend's Cookbook and Guide to Using Real Food to Fight Cancer

Annette Ramke & Kendall Scott

Foreword by David Katz, MD, MPH

RUNNING PRESS
PHILADELPHIA • LONDON

Designed by Frances J. Soo Ping Chow
Edited by Jennifer Kasius
Food stylist: Debbie Wahl
Prop stylist: Mariellen Melker
Typography: Aire, Bodoni, Lobster Two, Mr. Moustache Dingbats, and Neutra

Running Press Book Publishers
2300 Chestnut Street
Philadelphia, PA 19103-4371

Visit us on the web!
www.runningpresscooks.com

All those who have faced a major life challenge
and kept moving forward with determination,
because they just have way too much living left to do.

Our husbands,

who provided amazing support throughout our cancer journeys.

Our children,

for whom we wish a healthy, happy and cancer-free life.

May you grow up embracing the power of real food and always love

cooking and dancing in the kitchen.

Contents

PART TWO: THE RECIPES

Foreword

Honestly, I did not want to write another book foreword. As I draft this, I have several book deadlines of my own hanging over my head. I should have said no. I wanted to say no. But I could not resist this book—and neither should you!

The personal story here is enough all on its own: Two women who have been through cancer themselves, have learned all they can about keeping it a fading memory in life's rear view mirror, and who are committed to paying that knowledge forward. It is moving, compelling, poignant and so very...human. It calls out to us with what is common in us all: fear, hope, vulnerability and...strength. Resilience, resolve and resourcefulness.

That would probably have done it, frankly (ladies, you had me at "hello"!)—but there is, in fact, much more to this story, and to this book.

We have truly dramatic evidence of the potential power of food as medicine. The word dramatic is, well, dramatic—but nothing less suffices.

In 1993, a paper entitled "Actual Causes of Death in the United States" was published in the *Journal of the American Medical Association* by Drs. William Foege and J. Michael McGinnis. McGinnis and Foege revealed the obvious we had all overlooked: The diseases we had long listed as the leading causes of death (heart disease, cancer, stroke, diabetes) are not truly causes. Diseases are effects. What we all really want to know is: effects of what?

The answers were readily available. Overwhelmingly, premature death and chronic disease were attributable to just 10 behaviors each of us has the capacity to control, and that list of 10 is, in turn, much dominated by just the top three—tobacco use, dietary pattern and physical activity level.

When Centers for Disease Control and Prevention scientists reassessed this landscape a decade later, again publishing their findings in the *Journal of the American Medical Association*, in 2004, they found relatively little had changed. Across the span of a decade, injudicious use of feet, forks and fingers remained the dominant determinants of unwelcome fate.

In the summer of 2009, yet another paper was published by Centers for Disease Control and Prevention scientists and their colleagues—in the *Archives of Internal Medicine* this time—examining lifestyle factors and health. The investigators surveyed over 23,000 German adults about four behaviors: smoking (yes or no); eating well (yes or no); getting regular physical activity (yes or no); and maintaining a recommended weight (yes or no).

Those with all good answers—not smoking, eating well, active and lean—as compared to those with all bad answers had roughly an 80 percent lesser likelihood of experiencing any major chronic disease (cancer included). Flipping the switch from bad to good on any one of the factors was associated with a 50 percent reduced probability of chronic disease. Any drug with a faction of such potential would be a blockbuster. A group of researchers from Norway and England found much the same thing in a study of over 5,000 adults in the United Kingdom, reported in the *Archives of Internal Medicine* in April 2010; and researchers in the United States identified much the same pattern in a cohort here, reporting their findings in 2011.

The compelling case for feet, forks and fingers as the master levers of medical destiny reaches further still. In fact, it reaches to our very genes.

In a study reported in 2008 in the *Proceedings of the National Academy of Sciences*, 30 men with early stage prostate cancer received an intensive lifestyle intervention for 3 months: wholesome, plant-based nutrition; stress management; moderate exercise; and psychosocial support. Standard measures—weight, blood pressure, cholesterol and so on—all improved significantly, as one would expect. But what makes this study unique and groundbreaking is that it measured, using advanced laboratory techniques, the effects of the intervention on genes. Roughly 50 cancer suppressor genes became more active, and nearly 500 cancer promoter genes became less so.

This, and other studies like it, go so far as to indicate that the long-standing debate over the relative power of nature versus nurture is something of a boondoggle, for there is no true dichotomy. We can, in fact, nurture nature.

And it is to that very mission that *Kicking Cancer in the Kitchen* is devoted. The book dishes out a bounty of sound advice. But most importantly, as the title implies, it goes beyond advice to provide the ingredient-by-ingredient, user-friendly, practical guidance of recipes. This book is serving food, delicious food, as very powerful medicine.

I could not resist the compelling allure of this book. And whether you are recovering from cancer, or simply trying to make sure you never need to be—I suggest you not even try. Food is being served here as the very best of medicine, and I urge you—take it!

—David L. Katz, MD, MPH, FACPM, FACP
  Director, Yale University Prevention Research Center
  President-Elect, American College of Lifestyle Medicine

Introduction

If you've picked up this book chances are that you or someone you know has been affected by cancer. Having been there ourselves, we know what it's like when the shit hits the fan. Or when the fear of the C-word sends waves of worry throughout your still healthy body. Whether you are joining us after receiving a diagnosis, or are eager to learn all you can to stay disease free, we invite you to take us along on your journey to greater health and wholeness.

We wrote this book because we care about you. And we want to share with you, friend to friend, how to make a difference in your health and your life. Yes, you can do it! And we're here with a hug and a hand to walk alongside you. We'll do our best to help you embrace hope, enjoy a few laughs and create some tasty, cancer-kicking treats.

Perhaps, most importantly, our intention is to offer motivation, knowledge and a sense of empowerment to you, dear cancer chick, and to you, dear prevention peep, as well as to any determined woman who won't give up. There's just way too much living left to do.

What's Kicking Cancer in the Kitchen All About and Who Should Read It?

KICKING CANCER in the Kitchen provides real-world tools in and out of the kitchen for the woman facing cancer, from diagnosis through treatment and beyond. There are over a hundred of our favorite recipes you can quickly turn to—recipes that are simple, yummy and, most of all, cancer kicking! You'll be introduced to new, healthy, delicious cancer-fighting foods without feeling overwhelmed. We offer honest advice and tips on traveling the cancer path, all from our first-hand experience.

Kicking Cancer in the Kitchen is also for you if you are one of the millions of individuals who has cancer in her biography but is no longer in active treatment. This book will help you learn how to stay healthy and increase your odds of avoiding another encounter with the disease. And it is also a resource for the millions who live with the fear that one day they will hear those dreaded words, "You have cancer," and want to do all they can to make sure it never happens. If that is you, this book provides recipes and accessible advice to keep your body healthy. You'll also gain insight into how to support your sisters and friends who are on the cancer journey.

Our hope is that this book will help save a bit of your sanity as we've brought together our collaborative cancer journey knowledge, tools and recipes—while keeping things simple—so you don't have to spend precious time and energy, as we did, pulling it all together.

Our Dietary Recommendations

ARE WE VEGETARIAN, vegan or what? Well, honestly we don't like using labels very much. Our walk and talk is more about focusing on real, plant-based food and less about forcing ourselves to fit in a box or be part of a dietary trend. We also don't believe that shame or guilt about dietary choices, past or present, is conducive to your health. We're not down with blaming anyone for causing her cancer, nor are we cool with the idea of filling your plate with an ideology instead of health-boosting food that nourishes your body, mind and spirit.

But if you must label our approach in this book, you could call it flexitarian with a focus on plant-based, whole foods. Flexitarianism is, in theory, a mainly vegetarian diet but does allow for some animal protein on occasion. For us the meaning of this approach is broader, and we use it to refer to the practice of becoming aware of your body and its needs at every stage in your life and responding with personally appropriate dietary decisions. We are all unique and have different needs at different times in our lives, especially during cancer treatment. If a little animal protein gives you some needed energy during your cancer fight or otherwise, we aren't going to scold you. In fact, we'll even commend you for figuring out what your body needs.

But we do strive toward and encourage the reduction or omission of animal foods. It's fine to do this step by step, if that is what works best for you and will help make the changes stick. We believe that this is a much more realistic approach to improving your diet anyway, especially if you are currently a big meat-and-potatoes gal—the idea of suddenly becoming vegan can seem very daunting and you may just not make any changes. We'd rather see you slowly reduce and crowd out animal products by focusing on adding in more real, plant-based foods than not make any improvements at all.

In this book, we provide steps to work toward that plant-based, whole foods goal. Yes, some people have drastically changed their diets overnight, but let's be honest: It ain't easy! If you want to take on that challenge, please go for it. But if you are someone who needs a more gradual approach with a little more flexibility, your Girlfriends aren't going to ditch you. In fact we'll take your hand and support you as you "upgrade" your diet step by step. As long as you are taking strides in the right direction with that real food, mostly plants goal in mind, you're going to make a huge difference in your health. And no worries—you don't have to forgo taste or feel deprived. Eating well can taste delicious. We'll show you how!

Who Are Annette and Kendall?

————wwwwww————

WE ARE TWO young cancer survivors who not only survived but learned to *thrive* throughout our cancer journey—from diagnosis through intense treatment and beyond.

We get it. We know what it is like to be stopped in your tracks by what seems to be a death sentence. And we know what it's like to awaken from the post-diagnosis, scared-shitless stupor and wonder, "What the heck do I do now?!" However, we didn't want to just slog our way through cancer: We also wanted to look and feel as good as possible while doing it. And we did.

Between the two of us we have had three cancer diagnoses and countless surgeries and chemotherapy treatments. We've felt scared, pissed off and alone (despite being surrounded by caring, loving people) and we've also jumped for joy and learned to live expansively. We've tested different foods and recipes when we were nauseous from chemotherapy or dealing with day after day of fatigue. We've cried when our hair first started falling out, and later we learned to laugh about it (and wear some pretty funky wigs!).

So yeah, we get it, and we aren't afraid to express a little anger and blunt honesty here and there. Don't be surprised if we use a few not-so-nice words like "sucks" and "shit" because, let's face it, cancer isn't a nice disease, and we just want to keep it real. Beyond our cancer repertoire, we've also pursued training and careers in health and nutrition to increase our professional knowledge and understanding of food and our bodies.

But really, health-coaching credentials aside, we're here as two girlfriends who learned, step by step, that what we put into our bodies has the power to change our lives. That simply getting in the kitchen and enjoying real, whole foods could rock our world. And, let us tell you, if we could do and experience that you can, too!

This is what *Kicking Cancer in the Kitchen* offers: support, love, field-tested recipes and advice from two chicks who have been there and know a whole lot about learning to love themselves, food and life, even with cancer.

How to Use This Book

-~~~~~~~-

WE HAVE ORGANIZED this book into two main sections: "The Girlfriend's Guide" (Chapters 1 to 8) and "The Recipes." Chapters 1 and 2 contain our personal cancer stories as well as lots of support, resources and connection for "Cancer Chicks" and "Prevention Peeps" alike. Chapters 3 and 4 introduce you to cancer-fighting foods you will want to get friendly with, as well as advice on how to find your personal food groove. We'll take your hand in Chapter 5 and show you how to make healthy changes to your diet and life, one step at a time. Chapter 6 is full of advice around eating—whether during treatment, in the hospital, or on the go. Chapter 7 provides helpful information on eating for support around specific needs and treatment side effects. And yes, it's okay for cancer chicks to cry and eat chocolate: Chapter 8 is all about taking care of yourself and getting the love and care you need. "The Recipes" section contains ten categories and over a hundred recipes so you can not only read about using real food to help fight cancer, but you can also get right in your kitchen and start with your next beverage, snack or meal.

Kicking Cancer in the Kitchen is a cookbook, a guide, an invaluable resource for navigating the often overwhelming, sometimes scary and occasionally joyous world of cancer, deliciously.

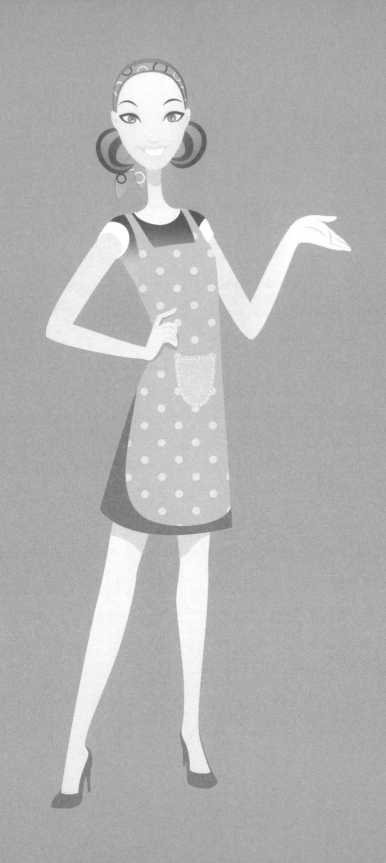

1

The Girlfriend's Guide

CHAPTER 1

It's a Whole New
(Cancer) World

Receive a cancer diagnosis and there it is, hanging overhead like a dark, foreign cloud. While your mind is trying to wrap itself around the meaning of this uninvited guest, sooner or later a few sparks begin to ignite: anger, love and fear. Anger at this horrible, unfair demon that has suddenly interrupted your life. Love of simply being alive and the overwhelming feeling that you're not ready to back out now. And fear. Fear is that interesting emotion that summons our fight or flight response. Give this choice to a woman who holds deep value for her own life and the happiness of those she loves most, and you end up with a chick ready for a fight.

There are some moments in life we'll always remember. Maybe it's the day you learned to ride a bike. Or received a much desired gift. Maybe it's the time you took your first jump off a diving board. Or that special someone said "I love you." Maybe it was the moment you realized there are no guarantees in life. Receiving a cancer diagnosis is undoubtedly one of those moments. Time seems to stand still as we hear the words we either feared or never expected to hear. Even writing about it now, at a distance separated by years, we can still feel that spot in our gut that took the punch and the cascade of emotions that accompanied it. Everything from shock, to silence, to utter sadness and fear, to—for some who may have been dealing with seemingly never ending tests and uncertainty—a feeling of strange relief to finally know what the heck is going on.

Welcome to Cancer World, a place no one willingly signs up to go, and where one thing is for certain: Life will never be the same. So when you wake up and find yourself in this heretofore alien place, it isn't hard to feel lost, scared and confused.

We know; we've been there, too.

Cancer World isn't a cool, juicy place where you hang out and sip drinks, a world in which everyone deals with the cancer crap like a champ and then lives happily ever after; it's fraught with decisions and loss and fear and, typically, its share of ugliness. So when you see us occasionally using some not-so-pretty words you'll know why—cancer isn't a pretty disease and sometimes we just need to tell it like it is. And so while we are here to empower and encourage you, and to help you get your groove back in cancer and in life, we never want you to think even for a minute that we don't remember just how rotten a place Cancer World can be. So know that we are always being friendly and never flip. And that we've got your back. 'Cause that's what girlfriends do!

Kendall's Story

WHEN I GOT the "You have cancer" phone call, I did four things in this order: I cried, I laughed, I drank a beer and ordered a pizza. I felt pure disbelief and shock, and my emotions were all over the place. But as I finished my greasy pizza and bottle of Stella Artois, I felt this ball of fortitude begin to form deep in my gut (and it wasn't just my dinner).

But let me back up to the beginning, at least, what I consider the beginning. I had been working for a few years in sales and marketing in the corporate world. It was the job I always thought I wanted and even though I worked very long hours, I felt like I had a position I could be quite happy with for a while.

Because of those long hours during the week, plus extra time on the weekends, I was overtired, stressed and didn't see my husband enough. I ate poorly, starting my day with a few cups of coffee, followed by a quick takeout lunch, some sweets for mid-afternoon snacks, and a late dinner that I put together quickly when I got home (or a pizza I had picked up on the way). I had no idea the toll this lifestyle was taking on my body. I paid no attention to the migraines, headaches and constant digestive issues I suffered from almost daily. I wasn't overweight, and I even fit in a workout a few times a week. And, believe it or not, I kind of liked my high-stress, coffee-and-sweets life.

So often, we measure our health by our weight, thinking that is the sole determining factor. And while, yes, weight is very important, it doesn't tell the entire story. People always told me I was lucky because I was tall and thin. Oh yeah, I was pretty lucky. I wasn't fat. Instead, I got cancer.

Things began to gain momentum one morning after I got to my office. I noticed some pain in my chest that hurt more with deeper breaths or if I sneezed or yawned. I had played a little golf early, before work, and thought perhaps I had pulled a muscle in my chest. The pain worsened over the course of the day and overnight it began to radiate down my right arm.

The next morning, I called my primary-care physician and they had me come in right away (apparently chest pain is nothing to laugh about!). After a few tests and my doctor deciding it wasn't my heart and that it probably was a pulled muscle, he was ready to send me home. As an afterthought, he mentioned having an X-ray taken, which I enthusiastically agreed to do. I just knew something wasn't right and that this was no pulled muscle.

The X-ray showed some sort of mass in the center of my chest, under my sternum, and my doctor thought it was just that my thymus gland was enlarged or that it could possibly be something with my heart, like an enlarged aorta. He consulted a specialist and based on his recommendation, ordered a CT (computed tomography) scan, which I had a few days later.

My chest CT showed a golf-ball sized mass that I was told was a tumor—*Wait! What?!*—but whether it was benign or malignant could not be determined at this point. My doctor told me the next step would be to have an abdominal and pelvic CT to find out if there were any other similar masses.

Waiting for the results of that scan was the longest couple of days of my life, and of my husband's. I kept thinking, okay, one malignant tumor in my chest I can handle. I can beat that. But if my insides were overrun with tumors? That I didn't know how to deal with. I remember going to a friend's birthday party with my husband the night after the abdominal scan and just feeling like I was walking around in a gray, ominous cloud. I was sick with fear and overwhelming dread. Everyone at the party seemed so far away, and all I wanted to do was snuggle up in my husband's arms at home.

A couple days later, we got the phone call that told us there were no other tumors found in the scans. That was the first good news we'd heard so far, and my husband and I both felt enormous relief! At that point, I was referred to a cardio-thoracic surgeon to make a decision on what to do about the tumor under my sternum. Because the mass was located so close to my heart, it seemed necessary for it to be removed whether or not it was malignant. Plus performing a biopsy in that location would be very difficult. Once removed, the mass would be biopsied. I was scheduled for major surgery: a full sternotomy. Oh yeah, that meant I was going to have my chest cut right open.

In surgery, they found that that "nasty tumor" (my surgeon's own words) had attached to the major vessels of my heart and my thymus gland and had wrapped around my right phrenic nerve, which is attached to the diaphragm. My surgeon was very aggressive in removing as much of the tumor as he could as well as my thymus gland. He also cut my right phrenic nerve to remove that part of the tumor, which left the right side of my diaphragm permanently paralyzed.

Recovering from this surgery was tough—the fracture in my sternum from opening up my chest would need eight weeks to heal. I was also trying to adjust to breathing with half a working diaphragm (fortunately the intercostal muscles surrounding that side learn to contract the diaphragm and make up for the phrenic nerve—our bodies are pretty amazing!). It was painful and I was exhausted. My surgeon said that kind of surgery is like being hit by a truck. He wasn't kidding. I slept a lot.

We waited about a week to receive the results of the biopsy from the tumor. I was feeling optimistic and kept telling myself there was no way it was cancer. When my surgeon called, he spoke with my husband first, and I could see it in his eyes as he listened to the doctor and looked at me. Cancer. Then I was handed the phone and got to hear those dreaded words myself. I scribbled "Hodgkin's lymphoma" and some other information down on a piece of scrap paper and hung up. That was when I cried, laughed, drank a beer and ordered pizza.

I have to say that no matter what happens with your cancer status, those initial moments stay with you. Writing this and reliving it three years later still brings tears to my eyes and a tightness in my chest. I will never forget the look on my husband's face, hearing "Hodgkin's lymphoma" and having no idea what that even was, or if I would be dead in a week. My mom was staying with us at the time to help me during recovery from surgery, and I can still hear her typing away on her laptop, most likely looking up information on Hodgkin's, while I cried in my husband's arms.

Then came the laughter, because I couldn't help but think how surreal this all was. Then I told my husband and mom that I didn't want to talk to anyone and that they could let the rest of our family know. I went up to our bedroom and sat in stunned silence (the beer and pizza came a little later). I acknowledged how terrified I was, and quickly accepted what this cancer may mean: death. And I was somewhat okay with that, or as okay as I could be. I had lived a wonderful twenty-seven years, and if my time was up, I thought I could come to terms with it.

My husband had different feelings about that. After giving me some time alone, he came to sit with me and told me I needed to fight this and that I couldn't give up. He made me promise that I would. I promised, although I didn't feel very confident about it.

What followed my diagnosis was a meeting with my oncologist and some tests, including blood work and a bone biopsy to determine how far along the cancer was. I also had a PET (positron emission tomography) scan. The only location the cancer seemed to be was in my chest area, and much of it had been removed through surgery. I was told I had stage IIa Hodgkin's lymphoma, nodular sclerosis, which is just the type of Hodgkin's. After discussing chemotherapy and radiation options, I opted for twelve treatments of ABVD (adriamycin bleomycin vinblastine dacarbazine) chemotherapy, which lasted about seven months. I had a medaport, or catheter, surgically implanted below my right shoulder, which was where my chemo cocktail would be administered. This, I was told, would help save the veins in my arms.

I won't lie: Chemo was tough. I went to the first treatment and was surprised that it wasn't as awful as I thought it would be. I left thinking, I can do this! It's not so bad! But it got much harder. My treatments lasted about four hours and I swear I could smell the drugs going into my medaport, which made me feel sick the entire time. I felt heavy, weak, exhausted, emotional and nauseous. Unfortunately, I also had a hard time sleeping, even though my body and mind were exhausted.

By my third treatment, I was dreading the drive to the treatment center, my hair was falling out in the shower and on my pillow and I had mouth sores that made eating painful. I had such anxiety, that I couldn't even say the word "chemo" when talking about my next treatment, and so my husband, a NASCAR fan, kindly referred to my treatments as "pit stops." After a couple more, I wanted to quit. I didn't think I could do it anymore.

It was during this time that I truly learned the meaning of "living in the moment" or being "mindful of the present." Anticipating my next treatment and the recovery time was so difficult and caused me so much anxiety, so I decided to focus on the time when I felt good. During my second week of recovery was when the intense chemo side effects seemed to subside, and I reveled in those moments and days of sweet relief. I didn't let my impending "pit stop" enter my mind. I got outside and got moving. I laughed with girlfriends. I took in deep breaths of fresh air. I spent the most wonderful moments with my husband. I learned to really appreciate my family, friends and people whom I didn't know so well, who offered me much needed support. I ran barefoot in the grass. I went skinny-dipping. I danced in my living room and sang at the top of my lungs in my car. And the more I focused on the moment I was in, the easier it became. I even learned to visualize these golden moments during the time I was in another chemotherapy treatment.

Before starting treatment, I had asked one of my cancer-team docs what else I could do to help fight this cancer. Should I eat certain foods? *Not* eat certain foods? I was told there was really nothing I could do. I didn't know then what I know now, but what I did know was that this doctor was wrong with a capital "W."

After a few chemo infusions, I began making some changes in my diet with help from my aunt, who is a health coach. I was eating more leafy greens and whole grains and cutting back on the processed foods and refined sugars. And, lo and behold, my recovery time between treatments shortened. I seemed to get my strength back sooner and wasn't quite as tired. My food gave me energy and it felt good knowing I was doing something to help my body. I even felt happier and more capable of handling my treatments.

This tremendous change motivated me to enroll in the Institute for Integrative Nutrition in New York City. I had only a few treatments left, but decided it was time to learn all I could about the importance of real, whole food and how it significantly affects our bodies. I wanted to make sure this cancer went away and never ever came back.

After completing the program in New York, I was a board-certified health coach, cancer-free and the healthiest and happiest I had ever been in my life. I knew I had the tools to continue listening to my body and to make the right choices in food and lifestyle, and to coach others in doing the same. I went into Cancer World sick, stressed and completely off balance, and came out of it with a fresh new outlook on food and life. (Not that it's quite that simple—you don't find out you're cancer-free and suddenly move on with your life like nothing happened and everything is all sunshine and rainbows. The time after graduating from active cancer treatment can be filled with its own challenges.) Still, overall, I was rejuvenated, grateful and totally psyched with my new food philosophy.

Annette's Story

————~~~~~~~~~————

THERE ARE TIMES in your life when, if you are listening closely enough, your body sends you signals that something isn't quite right. Maybe you develop aches and pains, can't sleep at all or sleep too much, or feel tossed and turned emotionally. Often we fail to notice these disturbances or, if we do, dismiss them for lack of time or chalk them up to "just the way life is." This was me in my early to mid thirties—busy with a young child and home, work and financial responsibilities. I didn't know I didn't have to feel that way.

As my body spoke louder and my intuition became stronger, I started looking for answers. A pain in my breast had me worried and I went from physician to chiropractor to talk therapist to try and figure it out. I also had a few friends in my life who had recently been diagnosed with breast cancer and, because of that, I started to really fear cancer and worry I might develop it, even though there was no history of breast cancer in my family.

After the various practitioners I was seeing provided only minimal relief, and were unanimous in their strong opinion that I was way too young to have to worry about breast cancer, I began to think it might just all be in my head. Thankfully my body kept shouting, and I found myself one day in the office of a breast specialist at a large university hospital. Although she too thought it would be unlikely I would have breast cancer, she took me and my concerns seriously and sent me for a mammogram. The test came back clear and I was relieved—although only somewhat, since I was still suffering from the symptoms I had been watching for quite a while now.

The specialist kept tabs on me regularly and all was well, until one evening when I noticed a slight change in my breast, which caught my attention. Trying to follow the advice my therapist had given me to "think horses, not zebras when you hear hoof beats" I thought I should probably just ignore it. Thankfully, something inside of me was wiser, and I saw myself going to the phone and calling for an appointment to run this new development past the breast specialist.

She wanted to see me, but insisted I get a current mammogram before the appointment. I **so** didn't want to go through that discomfort again and thought about just bailing on the appointment, figuring I was making a big deal out of a change so minor that even my husband couldn't quite see what I was noticing. Again thankfully, I found myself headed to the specialist's office with a pit stop beforehand at the imaging center for a fresh mammogram. The pit stop turned into the beginning of the nightmare I had always feared.

After taking the initial pictures, the technician called me back for additional images (these were the days before I turned every diagnostic test into a psych-out-the-tech game, looking for any possible overt or subtle sign as to whether to expect good news or the worst) and then, after what seemed like an eternity, a discussion with my doctor who, while encouraging me to keep hope and not freak out, said the images warranted a biopsy due to a suspicious potential malignancy. I was thirty-six years old.

As anyone who has been in this space knows, the days of waiting for tests and then for results are the longest days of your life. A radiologist performed the needle core biopsy in a dark room a week later, with my husband holding my hand and my heart beating through my chest. I asked her what her sense was and she told me that, while she had been wrong a handful of times in her career, she felt pretty certain this was cancer. Her phone call a few days later confirmed the suspicion and sent me through a wormhole and into a world out of which I would emerge forever changed.

Suddenly life stood still and, between bouts of silence and sobbing, apathy and anger, I resolved to do all I could to kick this disease and hopefully see my daughter grow up. I spent the following weeks discovering and exploring any option that came my way for fighting cancer. I looked at everything from off-the-wall alternative to completely conventional approaches, leaving my head spinning and my spirit pleading for wisdom and guidance.

Although I felt the pressure to move forward and make a decision, I allowed myself the time necessary to feel at peace with whatever decision I was going to make. Acknowledging my nature and my need to feel I was fleshing out all my options was important to me. This was the beginning of my journey into what would become an integrative approach to my cancer treatment—I just wasn't aware of that yet.

I decided there was wisdom in physically removing the tumor from my body, and scheduled a lumpectomy with my breast surgeon. The day of the surgery was probably one of the most traumatic in my whole life. I survived by feeling the love and support of all of those around me being sent strongly my way. Luckily the tumor was still relatively small and the nurse told me I would be up and out and on my way once it was removed. How wrong she would be.

It turned out my breast cancer had a nasty pathology and so I was sent to see an oncologist following the surgery. I had thought this would be a step I could avoid and was completely and utterly devastated. Luckily for me, I landed in the hands of not only an amazing breast oncologist but also a top researcher on genetics and cancer. Due to my young age, along with my pathology, she encouraged me to consider genetic testing. Although there had been no breast cancer in my family—which had led doctors before my diagnosis to conclude my risk for cancer was close to null—I did have a maternal aunt who had died of ovarian cancer, a possible sign of a genetic connection. It was clear to me that the more information I had the better, and I went ahead and took the simple blood test. It came back confirming my oncologist's hunch that I was positive for a mutation of the BRCA1 gene, one of the so-called "breast cancer genes."

It was recommended that I receive an aggressive course of chemotherapy along with an additional year of another intravenous chemotherapy drug specific to my type of cancer. From that point on visits to the chemo treatment center became a regular event for me for the following fifteen months.

At that point I began building my holistic cancer-kicking toolbox. I became immersed in conventional cancer treatment as well as nutrition—using food as medicine—and other healing modalities including everything from massage to meditation. I moved my body nearly every day, spent time in silence, accepted the support of friends, and filled my plate with cancer-kicking foods. And to my own amazement and the amazement of everyone around me, I started feeling better, looking brighter and enjoying life more than I ever had before—while in Cancer World!

I went for treatments. My hair fell out. I experienced pain and sadness. I had moments of joy and lightness. Life went on. Only it wasn't life as I had known it. It wasn't just a change, it was a metamorphosis. Physically, mentally, emotionally and spiritually I am a different person than I was B.C. (before cancer).

I mention this because at first, when we are hit with the cancer card, we naturally resist and want to hold on tightly to both the inside and outside manifestations of our lives. While it can be important to retain elements of your identity and life that you feel are essential or do not wish to part with, the ride in Cancer World can become less of a struggle when we practice the often challenging art of letting go. Letting go can happen more easily when it is not something we try to force but is rather something we cease to have a reason to resist.

Faced with my genetic status and the high likelihood my cancer could return, I made the very difficult decision following breast cancer treatment to have prophylactic bilateral mastectomies in the hope I could cease to be a patient forever and get on with the rest of my life. Cancer, however, had other plans for me.

After a long year and a half of breast cancer treatments and surgery, I gave myself the summer off. But not before, having just turned thirty-eight, I scheduled the prophylactic oophorectomy my oncologist had recommended, again due to the genetic mutation I carry. Little did I realize that, after just leaving Cancer World, I was about to be thrown back into it again.

My physicians were incredulous but were forced to bring me the news that malignancies had been found in my ovaries and fallopian tubes. As I listened to the surgeon's words on the telephone, I fell into a deep state of shock and disbelief. As my husband looked on, I began shaking my head No, uncontrollably. I couldn't do this again. I wouldn't do this again. Then my ten-year-old daughter walked over to me, had me make a tough, fighter face and pump up a muscle with my arm. She reminded me that I am strong and would fight this cancer just like I did the first one.

The bad thing about getting cancer twice is getting cancer twice. The good thing about it is you have been there before and, as much as it stinks, you know the ropes and have systems in place that make it all a teeny-tiny bit easier. I continued to build and tweak my integrative cancer-kicking toolbox. More surgery and chemotherapy (yes, I lost my hair again) came while I kept improving my diet, working on personal growth issues and moving my body when I could. I spent the long winter months of treatment curled up on my red couch for hours each day, often feeling lonely and weak but also experiencing peace and wondering what other lessons this journey had in store.

Fast forward to the present and you'll find a healthy young woman who survived cancer not once but twice and feels stronger and more vibrant in all aspects of her life than she ever felt before. The time when you leave Cancer World has its own challenges (and, we'd say, that's a whole other book . . . !) but I have emerged, ironically, more whole a person than I was when I went in, even though so much of "me" was lost to cancer.

I am convinced that the integrative approach I took both times to my cancer experience was the reason I was able to move through the grueling surgery, treatments and emotional havoc of the disease without any permanently devastating side effects, and with a strength and radiance which completely astonished and inspired those around me. It also led me to pursue further studies in nutrition and wellness coaching at the Institute for Integrative Nutrition in New York City. I am now a certified holistic health coach and work with those working on cancer prevention and recovery to help them learn that the kitchen is just as important as the pharmacy.

Cancer Is a Full-Time Job

- Making and going to doctor appointments.
- Dealing with insurance claims.
- Pleading to have pathology results forwarded—today!
- Managing the effects of treatment.
- Living with your cell phone constantly by your side,
  ready to grab at any moment of the day or night.

WHO KNEW HAVING cancer would turn out to be a full-time job? Oh, yeah, and then there's the rest of life, too: families, friends, work and other responsibilities. How to manage it all? It is definitely a challenging time when you first get hit with the cancer card: testing and waiting, sorting through and understanding the diagnosis, dealing with insurance companies and trying to find the proper physicians to consult with.

Finding Your Voice

A major source of personal growth for us during our time in Cancer World was being forced to find the strength of our voice and stand up and speak out on our own behalf. Sure we were modern women, successful in our school, work and personal worlds. Nonetheless, when faced with the emotions surrounding a potentially life-threatening illness, when dealing with strangers in white lab coats, and when feeling what seemed to be the weight of our world on our every decision, it was challenging to always muster the strength and confidence we needed to be our own best health advocate. While it can feel like a huge amount of pressure to decide how to approach cancer prevention, treatment or follow-up, it is not the time to stick your head in the sand (unless it means taking a trip to the beach to relax, in which case we'd suggest sticking your feet in the sand and not your head!). This is not the end of the road—there are options. Strengthen your voice and don't be afraid to use it. Seek out the support you need and look inside to find the wisdom that's in you to create the approach that is right for *you*.

Sometimes the "busy-ness" of the postdiagnosis period is a weird kind of blessing (it keeps you so busy you don't have much time to freak) and a curse (it is easy to feel like the rest of your life is determined by what happens in these days). Initially, it may be difficult to get in to see surgeons and other docs. But don't give up. Keep calling (be the squeaky wheel—a persistent but polite squeaky wheel!) and also get friendly with the scheduling staff and nurses. They often hold the key to getting you in faster for an appointment.

And remember, once you do get in to see Dr. Amazing, if you don't feel comfortable, keep looking. And even if you do feel great, sometimes getting a second opinion is a good idea. If for no other reason than to make you even more sure that opinion number one is really right for you. While it may feel like you need to take what you can get, remember that, in the end, doctors are working for you and should take the time to explain your diagnosis, your treatment options and, ideally, express openness to working with you and any other members of your Cancer Team (see below).

Prioritizing your efforts is the key here. It is easy to get overwhelmed when looking at the big picture. You are getting a lot of stuff thrown at you and it can seem like too much to process at times. Figure out what needs to be done first, and put your efforts into that. Once that is accomplished, move on to the next small step. And while some decisions do need to be made fairly swiftly, often there is time to weigh options and consider alternatives. Don't allow yourself to feel pressured unnecessarily, either by yourself or others.

And as challenging as it is, do take time each day to do some non-cancer stuff. Take a walk, call a friend and tell her you want to chat about anything except the C-word, try out the breathing exercise we have for you here in this chapter. This *is* your full-time job right now, but don't forget to take a water-cooler break every now and then.

This is also the time to ask for help. We repeat: Ask for help. We know how uncomfortable it can feel to request a helping hand. Our automatic reaction to the interrogative "Let me know if I can help" that rolls so often off the lips of our family and friends is usually to just say "Okay, I will," with no intention of ever taking up the offer. And that's that. Then we try to manage Cancer Headquarters, get to our appointments and get some food on the table then wonder why we are feeling so bad and sad.

Find a friend who can help you through the insurance maze. Grab some peeps who will put together a meal-delivery service for treatment days. Take up the offer of your aunt or cousin or neighbor to drive you to your appointment or pick up your child from school so you can nap. Accept your boss's offer to work from home when you need to. You get the picture. And you know what the secret is? These people really *want* to help you. Think of how you have felt when you've heard of someone else's crappy news. Doing something for that person is actually a way we help *ourselves* feel better. So let them do it to help you, and help themselves in the process.

Decisions, Decisions

——⌇⌇⌇⌇⌇⌇⌇⌇——

IF THERE IS one feeling we remember from the beginning of our time in Cancer World it is the feeling of wanting to know what we should do. We're talking *exactly* what we should do. *"If you do A, B and C in this order and for this duration then you will successfully fight cancer and live happily ever after..."* That's really not too much to ask, is it?

And initially we were willing to consider *anything*! Did someone read about a person who traveled to the Amazon, did handstands every day for a month and drank a special berry juice, and their tumor disappeared? Get us on the next flight!

Just Breathe

If cancer is detected in our body, the news itself can raise our anxiety level tremendously. Then, typically in quick succession, we prepare to undergo surgery and are given a debilitating course of chemotherapy and/or radiation. What could be more frightening? How are we to relax in the midst of the most stressful thing that has ever happened to us? How can we bypass the anxiety and despair that cause us to tighten up and turn away from life, and learn to recognize and pursue more positive possibilities?

Most of us are so used to being tense that we are not even conscious of our tightness. We tend to often unknowingly hold our breath or breathe very shallow. So start by just breathing! To focus more on your breathing try this exercise, called the Alternate Nostril Breath: Press the thumb of your right hand gently on the right side of your nose, plugging the nostril as you inhale slowly through the left nostril. Then place the ring finger of your right hand on the left side of your nose, plugging that nostril while releasing the thumb and the right nostril. Exhale through the right nostril. Then inhale through the right nostril, releasing your ring finger and left nostril as you plug your right nostril once again with your thumb. Exhale through the left nostril. Then inhale through the left, and continue to repeat this cycle for a total of 5 to 10 cycles.

Do our doctors suggest we take the most aggressive form of treatment and then we will have a whatever-percent chance of never encountering the Big C again? Get us to the hospital!

Take the traditional or an alternative approach, employ Eastern or Western medicine, pop pills or plead with prayer . . . we sometimes felt like we would literally burst if someone couldn't or didn't tell us the magic secret about what we needed to do to get through cancer and get on with our lives. Well, sometimes that wasn't a problem—opinions and advice about what to do abound. And sometimes we feel so much pressure to take a certain path that we don't even fully allow ourselves to realize that there are other approaches.

But what we wanted was a fail-proof, 100 percent guaranteed-to-kick-cancer's-ugly-ass plan. And besides, our minds were so busy with all the angst surrounding the diagnosis, where were we supposed to get the brain power to not only consider but *find* all of our options?! And then the whole matter of having to take responsibility for our decisions? Crap! Can someone else take over that part?! Will I regret not doing A? Should I do B and then A? My girlfriend did C and it didn't go well. But so-and-so did D and she has been cancer-free for ten years.

Talk about feeling overwhelmed and scared and anxious and angry and impatient. It's the worst! The upside to all this is the fact that, in most cases, this isn't the end of the road. There are almost always options. Embracing your inner core of strength and motivation will help you put the pieces of your personal Kicking Cancer Plan together, bit by bit.

It's important to remember that cancer is not personal—the disease is not out to get just you—and that anyone can get hit with a diagnosis at any time. But cancer treatment is personal—it will be unique to you and your cancer. This means that there's no need to compare yourself to others, or to some "standard" for what decisions you are making and how you are doing and feeling. There is no one-size-fits-all in life, and that includes cancer prevention and treatment.

Beyond treatment-related decisions, there are a host of other ones related to managing the rest of your life while in Cancer World. One we want to mention is the decision about with whom to share your cancer status and how much of your story you want to share. There is no one right answer (big surprise!) to this question. The important thing here is to go with what makes *you* feel comfortable. If you feel better only letting a few close people in your life know, that's fine. And if it helps you to chat about what's going on with everyone in your family and social circle, that's okay, too. Don't feel pressured either way to share less or more than what feels right to you and be sure that those around you respect your decision.

If you do want to keep anywhere from a few to a slew of people up to date on your journey through cancer, a couple of helpful resources are Care Pages (www.carepages.com) and Caring Bridge (www.caringbridge.com). At these web sites you can set up an account and post news which gets sent out to anyone who has signed up to receive your updates. This saves writing a bunch of individual messages and lets everyone you want to keep in the loop know how you are doing.

Decisions also abound when you have completed active cancer treatment as well as when you are placing a priority on prevention. How much testing is the right amount? Should you put your trust in drugs or diet (or both)? Where do you place the focus in your life now?

That being said, we can't say enough about the importance of stepping up to the plate, making the best decision possible with the knowledge and insight you have at the moment, and then not second-guessing yourself or looking back. Just keep putting one foot in front of the other and move forward. Look inside and you will likely find strength you didn't know you had, and the resolve to take this shitty disease and kick it as hard as you can.

What Else Can I Do? Integrate!

———〰〰〰〰〰———

WE'RE BOTH INCREDIBLY thankful for modern medicine and for our MDs and nurses who helped us on our journey through cancer. The diagnostic tools they use and the cancer treatment options they gave us fall under the category of "conventional medicine," which is the kind of medicine one encounters in most hospitals and doctors' offices today.

Conventional medicine has its place—we can't imagine suffering a life-threatening accident or sustaining major trauma and not being grateful for its tools. And most cancer chicks, including us, choose to use some combination of surgery, chemotherapy, radiation and other cancer treatments that Western medicine offers.

For us, a huge part of our empowerment around cancer came through being forced into the situation of having to evaluate our diagnosis, and then exploring options and putting together the best Cancer Team we could possibly find. We began by looking at conventional medicine options and branched out from there to explore other approaches.

You may have heard of the term "alternative medicine." What does that mean? Alternative medicine is medicine used *instead of* conventional medicine. If used in combination with conventional medicine, you'll hear it referred to as "complementary medicine." We became convinced of the wisdom of combining the best of conventional and the best of complementary and alternative medical (or CAM, for short) approaches to cancer treatment into an *integrative* cancer-kicking program. Integrative refers to a combination of mainstream medical therapies and CAM.

Rather than marry ourselves to a specific ideology or approach, we looked at the disease and our life as a whole and decided to tackle it with our newfound holistic toolbox. At first the toolbox was pretty empty. But as we learned more and explored options, we continued to add to it.

Sometimes we would place a tool in the box, but it didn't really fit right or help much, and we took it out. Toolboxes can be tweaked. Sometimes we would grab a tool and throw it in the box because a friend of a friend recommended it to us as *the best tool ever*, but it didn't do the job for us. Toolboxes must be personal. And then, one day on our cancer journey, we looked into our toolbox and had that feeling that Goldilocks had when she sat in Baby Bear's chair: just right!

What will you put in your cancer-kicking toolbox? (We'll give you lots of ideas throughout the book.)

We want to give you the low-down on some of the members of our Cancer Team—an integral part of our cancer-kicking toolbox—who may be less familiar to you. They are all great to have on board whether you are in active treatment or want to strengthen your body to avoid the disease. Take a look and see if they might be a good addition to your lineup.

Naturopaths

NATUROPATHIC MEDICINE USES natural substances and treatments to support the body and its ability to heal. The primary goal of naturopathic treatment is to address the *cause* of illness, rather than simply treat or suppress *symptoms*. A naturopathic doctor (ND) spends a significant amount of time with the patient and sees her as a whole person, taking into account the physical, mental, emotional and spiritual dimensions when diagnosing and developing a treatment plan.

Naturopathic doctors take four years of premedical, undergraduate studies, followed by four years at a college of naturopathic medicine that includes a standard medical curriculum along with complementary modalities. Currently, sixteen states, the District of Columbia and the U.S. territories of Puerto Rico and the Virgin Islands have licensing laws for naturopathic doctors. In these states, naturopathic doctors are required to graduate from an accredited four-year residential naturopathic medical school and pass an extensive postdoctoral board examination (NPLEX) in order to receive a license.

Naturopaths can support cancer chicks using nutrition, supplements, homeopathy, herbal medicine and lifestyle coaching during treatment, including surgery, chemotherapy and radiation. They are also ideal partners for those recovering from treatment or those individuals focusing on cancer prevention and overall health.

Acupuncture

ACUPUNCTURE BELONGS TO the system of Chinese medicine that dates back to as far as 3000 BCE. While acupuncture is the most often practiced component of Chinese medicine (CM), it is simply that: a component, an important piece of a much larger practice. Along with acupuncture, CM employs other techniques such as acupressure, moxibustion, herbal medicine, diet and lifestyle changes and meditation.

According to theory, there are as many as two thousand acupuncture points on the human body, connected by twenty pathways called meridians. These meridians conduct qi (pronounced *chi*) between the surface of the body and the internal organs. Qi, a concept emphasized in Chinese medicine that has no true counterpart in Western medicine, is considered a vital force or energy and is thought to help regulate balance in the body. Acupuncture is believed to normalize the flow of qi throughout the body and support the restoration of health to the mind and body.

If you are going through cancer treatment and the thought of more needles makes you feel like running in the opposite direction, don't dismiss acupuncture too quickly. Unlike hypodermic needles, acupuncture needles are solid and hair-thin and are not designed to puncture the skin. They are also inserted to much more shallow levels than hypodermic needles. While each person experiences acupuncture differently, most feel very little discomfort as the needles are inserted.

Look for an experienced acupuncturist who has passed state and national license exams and has worked with a significant number of cancer chicks. Some practitioners even have qualifications from cancer hospitals such as Sloan Kettering where they have studied specific protocols for use during cancer treatment. These acupuncture protocols can be a big help with issues such as nausea, low blood counts and neuropathy.

Kendall:

I saw an acupuncturist during chemotherapy to help reduce nausea and anxiety and rebalance my body. My appointments were relaxing and I hardly felt the little pricks from the needles. It's definitely worth trying out and may become a key part of your cancer toolbox.

Integrative MDs

IT IS RARE for our traditional MDs to take a holistic view of us or the cancer. Their approach is generally based pretty directly on the test-diagnose-treat method. Here's where having an integrative MD on your team can be a huge advantage. He or she looks at us as a whole person—body, mind and spirit—as well as considering a wide range of factors in life that can influence health, wellness and disease. Integrative MDs then create a partnership between themselves and their patients and make use of both conventional and complementary alternative methods to support the body's natural healing response. They focus on therapies which are grounded in science while preferring the use of effective but less invasive options whenever possible. These docs embrace and teach self-care based on broader concepts of treatment and healing than their traditional MD counterparts. They can provide support with everything from guidance in choosing conventional treatment options to selecting appropriate and effective complementary tools such as vitamins and other supplements, mind-body practices and diet and lifestyle recommendations.

We found great strength and confidence in knowing we had a group of amazing health care professionals who together covered all the bases in our holistic, integrative approach to cancer treatment. Knowing we had people who did their jobs well, were on top of our situation, communicated with each other, and gave us the feeling of really caring about us helped us on a physical and psychological level together to pull through. That team, together with our discovery of the power of real food to heal and strengthen, helped us to not only survive but thrive through cancer treatment, and beyond.

Annette:

The integrative MD I worked with during cancer treatment had effective, natural tools, like supplements, dietary guidance and visualization techniques, for supporting me during cancer treatment and recovery. Beyond that he collaborated with my oncologist to add some additional elements to my chemotherapy regimen to help prevent nasties like neuropathy (a numbness or tingling in hands and feet as a result of nerve damage) and nausea. He also checked up on important stuff like making sure my vitamin D levels were adequate and that I was getting myself on my meditation cushion regularly.

The Nutrition Link: Real Food Changes Everything

ON OUR JOURNEY through Cancer World we were both fortunate enough to become acquainted with the power of real food. While we both would have said, pre-cancer, that our diets were pretty good—we rarely ate fast food, didn't slurp sodas and tried to eat our vegetables—once we began studying the connection between food and disease, we learned that our assessment of what we were putting into our mouths and bodies was—umm—a bit off base. Delving into the nitty-gritty of nutrition, as well as training with whole-foods chefs and spending gobs of time in the kitchen, we both came to experience firsthand just how much real food can completely change everything.

We went from takeout pizza and meat and potatoes to leafy green veggies and whole grains in baby steps, and as we did, we felt the improvement. Our energy drastically increased, digestive issues subsided, our skin acquired a glow and our moods evened out. Oh right, and this was all while we were undergoing intense chemotherapy and recovering from major surgery. From our own experience we can assure you that eating real, plant-based food can help you feel better physically and be stronger psychologically—with or without cancer.

Frame Your Focus

Cancer survivors, us included, often speak about fighting cancer. This is, of course, because we all hate cancer and work and wish for the day that this horrible disease is no longer able to harm us. Though the idea of embracing the fight can be powerful and galvanizing, we've also found that the moments we are able to envision what we *do* want—health, physical and mental well-being—rather than on what we *don't* want—cancer—we feel even stronger and more peaceful. For example, you might try creating a personal, positive affirmation such as "Every day in every way my body is getting healthier." Or "I am brave, strong and full of life. My body, mind and spirit are in balance." As hard as it can be, especially immediately post-diagnosis, we would encourage you to try this approach to framing your focus and see if shifting your thoughts from what you *don't* want to what you *do* want makes a difference.

In a society in which time is money and food is merely fuel to keep your body up and running (or an emotional crutch to soothe and satisfy), we typically fail to make the connection between what we put into our body and how we feel. We also neglect to place any importance on taking the time and making the effort to learn about healthy eating and preparing and consuming nutrient-rich, disease-fighting meals.

The secret to health can be found in the saying we've heard so often that we fail to recognize its wisdom: *"You are what you eat."* Food is a key factor in determining if we stay healthy or develop disease, feel energized or worn out, embrace hope or drown in depression. All of these areas in our life and more are fueled by our food— and we often thoughtlessly throw something down our throat to quiet the hunger.

Interestingly enough, cancer as well as almost any disease, is highly linked to the food we eat, our surroundings and stress, and can be simplified even more when we break it down into two components: deficiency and toxicity. When you eat poorly, your body is not getting the nutrients it needs, so deficiencies arise and the body is not able to effectively disarm toxins. This, in turn, creates an environment in which our bodies cannot function properly, fight off disease or heal as they should. By cleaning up our diets and creating a healthier lifestyle, we are able to alleviate deficiencies and remove toxins so the body can carry on its intrinsic healing process.

When we are suddenly faced with a cancer diagnosis, or want to do all we can to prevent the disease in the first place, realizing that what we put in our mouths impacts the quality and, very likely, quantity of our life is empowering. Suddenly there is something more we can do. You aren't just cooking dinner anymore: You are caring for your body. Overnight the kitchen ceases to be a dreaded place but rather is transformed into a sacred space. And real food is not something we are scared of but becomes our best friend.

Taking the leap out of the familiar grocery-store aisles lined with cans and boxes and instead filling our shopping carts and our plates with fresh whole food is the way to create strength, health and well-being, whether you're living with cancer or not.

Because of the amazing changes we have witnessed in ourselves and our clients, we are convinced of the power of real food to change everything and can't wait to share our knowledge and experience with you throughout this book. Whether you are cooking for yourself, or having others do it for you, we'll show you exactly what we did and how we did it. (You can jump ahead to Chapter 3 and beyond if you can't wait.)

So, dear girlfriend, we are here to share a hug, to let you know you can make it, and to join you, step by step, as you transition to a healthier diet and a happier, more amazing life.

CHAPTER 2

Sharing the Journey

One of the positive aspects about having gone through cancer ourselves is that we can share some of our experience with you. We can even talk about the things that no one really wants to talk about, but that are still there. So often, when you're going through this stuff for the first time, it's tough to find someone to talk to who really gets it and who can say, "Yeah, that totally stinks" or "I know! Isn't that an awful feeling?" Sometimes it's just nice to have a fellow cancer chick validate what you may be feeling. And remember, whatever you may be feeling about your cancer status—whether prevention, treatment or recovery—is totally okay. Don't be afraid to own your feelings and thoughts surrounding this crazy ride. There is no right or wrong way to feel, behave or think.

More Than a Label

WHEN YOU RECEIVE a cancer diagnosis, suddenly you are whipped into the world of cancer where there is a name for everything, including you. Before you may have been, "Suzy Jones, mom of two, teacher," but now that description seems to virtually disappear and your title unwillingly becomes "cancer patient" or "cancer survivor." This is what you are in your doctor's office or many cancer support groups, which may make sense, but it still gives you a definition you may not be comfortable with.

Even family, friends, coworkers and others who hear of your diagnosis through the grapevine may find it hard not to label you as "the girl with cancer." Then there are the assumptions that seem to go along with it: sick, bald, dying . . . dead? And can you blame these labels and assumptions? Hey, before we got cancer and learned what it was all about and what it felt like to be in those shoes, we really had no clue and probably thought the same things. Cancer is a big scary unknown to a lot of people, and it's difficult to know the proper etiquette. And maybe that's because there is none.

If you don't want to be labeled as a "cancer patient," call yourself something else. Cancer chick, cancer crusher or cancer ass-kicker—okay, we are just being silly, but seriously, do whatever it takes to make this time easier and even a tad humorous. Or ditch the label and don't call yourself anything at all. Sometimes we find ourselves simply saying in conversation, "I went through the cancer stuff myself" instead of, "Why yes, I am a cancer survivor." See the difference there? It places cancer as a part of your life and a part of you instead of making it *all* of you (although we know that it can certainly feel that it *is* your entire life when you're right in the thick of it).

It can be too easy sometimes to play the part of the label we are automatically given with a cancer diagnosis, and that begins to eat away at who we really are. It's important to try not to lose your identity to cancer, even when it's taking over your life and has become your full-time job. Find time in your day to do something that doesn't focus on cancer and how crappy and scared you feel. Yeah, we know it always seems to be looming over you anyway, but still, make some non-cancer time to help you remember (or try to figure out) who you really are, or to simply put the cancer aside.

You Don't Have to Like Pink

FOR MANY WOMEN being part of a local or national cancer-related movement offers support and connection and helps them to be proactive during their cancer journey. But like we've said, you don't have to be the poster girl for cancer. Don't feel the need to adorn yourself with cancer pins, T-shirts or get a bumper sticker if it's not your thing. Don't pressure yourself to join every fund-raising event around. There are some great causes out there, but getting involved isn't every gal's cup of tea. Be real with yourself and use this time to feel what you want to feel, act how you want to act, and get involved with whatever you want (or not).

Breast cancer support is the best example because we see the pink paraphernalia everywhere. You've probably seen the pink hats, ribbons, coffee mugs, bracelets, water bottles, pens, calendars, socks, home décor, teddy bears and so much more. For many women, sporting the pink gives them a sense of belonging, hope and courage, and that's fabulous. Many of the proceeds from sales from these items support worthy causes. However, if you do have breast cancer, do not feel obligated to sport your pink ribbon unless it feels right to you. We know some breast cancer babes who truly get sick of all the pink stuff, but they are still amazing women who are working through their cancer and supporting fellow cancer chicks and organizations at their own comfort level.

Beware of the pink promotions that seem to go a little too far. Remember the pink KFC bucket of fried chicken? We aren't sure how encouraging people to purchase and eat a bucket of factory-farmed chicken cooked in grease promotes good

Kendall:

My husband is the most wonderful, caring husband on this planet and during my treatment he was supportive and loving and did so much for me. The entire experience brought us closer and our marriage really grew and flourished as a result. However, there were still times when I felt a little lonely. I kept thinking how fortunate I was to have such amazing support, but at the same time I thought sadly to myself, no one *really* gets it. I had all these mixed emotions and it seemed that no matter what I did some days, that cancer just loomed over me, just to make sure I didn't forget about it. As if I could.

health. Anyone fighting breast cancer or trying to prevent it should probably avoid those buckets and support breast cancer organizations in other ways.

Think Before You Pink (see Resources; page 320) is a project of an organization called Breast Cancer Action. This project was launched as concern grew around the increasing number of pink ribbon products on the market. The project's mission is to hold companies more accountable for their pink ribbon promotions and to encourage consumers to do their research and find out who or what a pink ribbon product benefits. It's important to be aware of who is funding different cancer campaigns, some of which include pharmaceutical companies or other businesses that benefit from higher rates of cancer or actually create products that promote cancer itself. The point is, be a savvy consumer and know what that ribbon is representing and who actually profits from the sale.

Stupid Lonely Cancer

IN CASE YOU hadn't noticed, cancer is lonely. You can have the most wonderful, supportive spouse or partner, parents, friends and children who would do anything to help you through this, but it's just not quite enough sometimes. Unless you've been thrown into Cancer World yourself, it's just impossible to completely grasp what it feels like. And that's understandable. It's kind of like giving birth. Until you've done it, you'll never quite get it. So, congratulations, you're giving birth to one heck of a watermelon.

And here's a little side note: As difficult as it might be while you're going through all your cancer stuff, try to remember that it's often just as hard on your loved ones. It's tough for them to not know how you're really feeling, and they can feel very helpless themselves seeing you sick or sad. While it's your job to focus on you right now, keep that in the back of your mind and don't forget to show them some love.

As we've gone through our cancer journeys, we remember having conversations with other cancer gals, and some referred to their cancer diagnosis as "going through the worm hole." Once you go in, you don't come back out the same way, and it's completely different on the other side. And that applies no matter what the future holds. Even when you are cancer-free for years, it's still there. It's always a part of you, for better or for worse. Oh, that crappy cancer.

Okay, so it's friggin' lonely. That's the problem. Here is a possible solution: Find other people who have been through it or who are going through it now. Listen to their experiences. Talk about yours. It's amazing how much that connection helps the loneliness fade away, or at least seem more bearable. You'll see that you aren't the only one who's feeling alone and scared.

There are many cancer support groups out there, so don't be afraid to check them out. If you aren't into the group thing—which we get, sometimes we like to go solo, too—check out cancer web sites with message boards, forums, blogs and social media like Twitter. You'd be amazed at how much support you can find online from others who have had or currently have cancer. They will share their stories, fears, questions and accomplishments. What's nice about these virtual support systems is that you can still remain pretty anonymous, if that's more comfortable to you. Whether you decide to try the in-person group scene or prowl on some cancer-support message boards, don't be afraid to put yourself out there and find out what is available to you. Once you do, you will begin feeling a whole lot better.

Remember when we said that cancer is a part of you, for better or for worse? Well, fortunately, the "better" can be easier to find than you may think. Yes, cancer is stupid and lonely, but many amazing, good things can come from it. It takes a little positive thinking, some self-motivation and that inner desire to transcend being a lonely soul and body with cancer.

This may mean simply reflecting over time on all that you have endured physically, emotionally and mentally and how it has changed you as a person. It could mean focusing on all that you do have to be thankful for. Sometimes all of the good in your life can really stand out when you've been in Cancer World, and sometimes you have to look for it. It could also mean supporting other cancer gals through different buddy programs, support groups or in the virtual realm. Here are some of the good and wonderful things that have come from our cancer experiences:

- The "bad" stuff that used to make us freak out (like a horrible haircut) doesn't seem *quite* as awful now. It's easier to let it go.

- When other people around us are newly diagnosed, we are able to offer some advice and even explain some of the medical jargon and procedures that they may be encountering. This helps to make it a little less lonely for that new cancer chick.

- We wrote a book to share our cancer stuff and to help you and others!

- We've changed our eating habits, which not only helped in fighting the cancer, but has also helped us to feel strong, ease digestive issues, get fewer colds and maintain a healthy weight.

- We discovered that getting in the kitchen and trying new foods is fun and inspiring.

- We are more compassionate toward others because you just never know what that person might be going through.

- We've learned the true meaning of and practice taking the time to "stop and smell the roses."

- The good relationships with people in our lives hold more value, and it's easier to know which relationships are worth strengthening or are just too draining to hold on to.

- The "quality versus quantity" concept seems to apply readily to everything. It's the quality of relationships, daily activities, food and life in general that matters, not the quantity.

We encourage you to take a little (or a lot) of time trying to determine the "good" that may have come from your cancer. Could it be an opportunity, rather than a horrible, traumatic experience? Could cancer be your personal teacher? Research has even shown that the people who try to find the silver lining on their cancer cloud are often happier and have a better chance of kicking the disease. Hey, that positive thinking stuff can really work!

Hair and There

FOR SOME WOMEN, losing their hair can be one of the scariest parts of cancer treatment. For many of us, our hair is part of who we are. So when we're suddenly given the Cancer Card and realize chemotherapy may be in the near future, that fear of hair loss comes crashing in. Not only do we have to fight crappy cancer, but now we have to feel ugly and embarrassed by thinning hair or no hair at all. Pretty unfair. And yeah, it may feel silly and vain in the grand scheme of things (okay, I'll lose my hair, but if it means I get to live, then it's worth it right?!), but still, it's tough to let go of our locks.

Hair Matters

If you need a little help finding head and hair accessories, try some of the web sites below. Also be sure to look for local resources. Start by asking for a referral from your treatment center or hospital. Also, be sure to check with your health insurance company, because wigs and head wraps are often covered with a note from your doctor.

www.softhats.com
www.headcovers.com
www.4women.com

Kendall's Hair Story:

When I started chemo, my hair was long, and I had worked for a few years to get it to that length. I decided, before I even lost any hair, to just have it cut into a chin-length bob. I figured it would be easier for me to handle losing shorter hair than hair that was almost 24 inches long. It first started falling out in the shower one morning. It came out in my hand. I had been anticipating the hair loss, but was still shocked to see it happen. I cried through the rest of my shower.

About a week and a half later, after I had been consistently losing hair little by little, I was walking with my friend from our car to a restaurant. It was a very windy evening, and I just couldn't help but see the humor in my situation and said, "I better put my hood on, or else this wind is going to blow my hair right off my head, and I can't afford to lose any more right now!"

Another couple of weeks went by and my hair got thinner. I made another appointment for a haircut and got it chopped right off into a short pixie cut, less than an inch long. When I first looked in the mirror, I told my husband, who had come with me to the appointment, "Great, I look like our nephews." Don't get me wrong, our nephews, who were ages four and six at the time, were and are wonderful, good-looking kids. But, come on. I didn't want to look like a 6-year-old boy.

My hair continued to fall out, but I never went completely bald. It was just noticeably thin. Very noticeably. I did get fitted for a wig, which I purchased, but I only wore it a few times. Most of the time I wore nothing on my head, or a hat on colder days. Oddly enough, I felt empowered and was even slightly happy that I didn't have hair to worry about for a little while. I saved plenty of money by not buying hair products! I did have my bad days when I felt ugly and sick-looking, but overall I was pretty okay with the hair loss. I kept reminding myself that I didn't need hair to laugh, have fun or enjoy the fresh air and sunshine outside. I didn't need hair to snuggle with my husband or go for a walk. It made me realize that my hair didn't make me who I was, and that was liberating. Plus, what could I really do about it? I couldn't really stop my hair from falling out or make it grow in faster. So I decided to accept it and move on. Once I finished chemo, my hair began growing again, and I was able to try new cute haircuts at different lengths as it grew in. And, I was shocked to find that I really liked my hair short. I would never have had the guts to chop it off if it wasn't for my impending hair loss, so in many ways, I'm glad I had the opportunity to try something new.

Whether or not you actually lose any hair and how much completely depends on the type of chemotherapy you receive, but most chemotherapy treatments will trigger at least a little hair loss. You can ask your oncologist what is typical for your treatment, but remember that everyone is different and you may lose more or less than the norm. Your chemo cocktail is most likely designed to slow down or eliminate rapidly replicating cells. Your hair is a fast growing cell, so it is usually affected in the process. Boo.

When that very first clump of hair falls out, it can be quite disturbing. It often comes out in the shower or you'll find a clump or a few strands on your pillow in the morning. You'll run your fingers through your hair only to find it coming out in your hand. And then there's more the next day, and the next. You may start to have bald spots, or it may thin evenly. For some women, it comes out slowly and for others it happens rather quickly.

Now hold on, don't panic! If you know that your hair may indeed fall out, it's nice to have a plan in place so you at least feel somewhat in control of the situation and your head. Here are options and ideas that may work for you, and that many women have used themselves (including us!).

- Before your hair actually begins to fall out, play around with scarves, hair wraps and hats to see what you like on your head. If you think you may want to wear a wig, try some on. You can do this on your own, but we suggest finding a hair salon in your area that carries wigs and works with cancer clientele. You should be able to get a referral from your treatment center. You may wish to purchase a wig and head wraps before your hair even comes out, just so you have something ready to wear. Many insurance companies will reimburse you for the cost of a wig—just ask your doctor to write a prescription for a cranial prosthesis.

- When those first few locks of hair fall out, get thee to the salon and have all your hair shaved off. Or, if your hair seems to be coming out slowly, get a shorter pixie haircut so it doesn't look so thin. Then have it shaved off later (or not).

- Shave your hair off at home when you are sick of seeing the locks of hair in your shower drain. Have a friend or family member assist and support you.

- Consider donating your cut hair to an organization like Locks of Love or the Childhood Leukemia Foundation so that others may benefit. Be sure to find out the donation specifications—some organizations require the hair to be a certain length or thickness.

Whatever you decide to do, remember that it is your choice, and yours alone. If you want to cover your head with a wig, wrap, hat or anything else, have fun with it! Try different styles and colors. Get some funky hats or stick with simple beanies that keep your head covered and warm. Find a leopard-print head wrap or just stick with a few nice colors. You could try to find a wig that closely resembles your natural hair, or use this opportunity to try out a new look (or a few!). And maybe you'll

Annette's Hair Story:

Getting hit with cancer twice meant—ugh!—going through the hair loss thing two times. The first time around I engaged in a lot of hopeful thinking —maybe I might be one of the rare individuals who would defy the odds of my chemo cocktail's side effects and wouldn't lose all of her hair. Unfortunately, that idea remained in the realm of wishful thinking!

I got a lot of well-meaning advice around losing my hair, most of which I found useful but some of which didn't ring true for me. I followed the suggestions to find a wig and some head wraps and hats before the hair headed out (pun intended). But I decided not to chop my (long, beautiful) hair off before it fell out. Everyone had been telling me it would make the transition easier. The thought, though, of having to adapt to and accept a short cut before losing it all seemed too much for me. I wanted to hang on to my long hair until the last possible moment. So I stood my ground and bided my time.

And then one day, when there was more hair in my hand than on my head, I went straight to my hairdresser (who kindly let me come in during off hours, so I could have privacy) to get shaved. I always felt I must be so vain for being so affected by my hair loss. Now I know, after talking to lots of other women, that it can indeed be a very traumatic event. No need to feel like you're superficial if you are down and out about your hair loss: It is a completely normal reaction and you are far from alone.

The first time I was in Cancer World it was super important to me to retain my pre-cancer identity. And a large part of my identity to the outside world was how I looked. Even though I was happy to have the support and concern of those around me, I also mostly just wanted to feel "normal" and not have anyone notice. I didn't want to have to deal with people seeing me bald and acting like I was *this close* to death. And I already felt outside of society with my diagnosis and the way some people and medical professionals treated me (me = cancer patient = sick = different).

So I found a wig that most closely resembled my natural hair color and length. This wig allowed me to feel comfortable and move about in the world without getting stares and sad looks as I got groceries, drove my daughter to activities or just took a walk in the neighborhood. It truly saved me emotionally and mentally. As tough as it was to lose my hair and don the wig, I grew to be able to make jokes about how my shower and bathroom time got slashed, and how I could just whip on my wig and look like I stepped out of the salon!

And it wasn't any easier the second time around. It seemed super unfair to have to lose it all over again. Although this time I wasn't as concerned about always looking like my "old self" (what was that now, anyway?), I did get a new wig and some pretty wraps. And thank goodness I had hung onto my favorite snuggly fleece cap to keep my little bald head from freezing during the night! This time I was fine presenting myself without any hair—real or not—and was able to feel more at ease with just a hat or a cool silk scarf. I definitely felt more comfortable and didn't fear the public glances and whispers that often accompany being an obvious "cancer patient." I also learned to play a bit and enjoyed a fun wig collection that a fellow cancer peep gave me for my bald time. And by the end of my treatment time I had become so empowered that I bought a beautiful, long white dress and went to a special place to have my picture taken as a gorgeous, bald goddess.

So you see, there is no right or wrong way to deal with the hair-loss thing. Find what works for you—everyone has her own comfort level and personal style. And, even though it may be hard at times, resist the urge to slap (as I wanted to) those well-intentioned non-cancer folk who tell you "it will grow back." Because—you know what?—it will.

feel like breaking out a hot pink wig for special occasions. These days, wigs look very realistic and can be adjusted to fit your head pretty perfectly so you don't feel like you're faking it.

Another possibility is to just bare that beautiful head. Some women choose to be bald and then play up the accessories, like earrings, necklaces or neck scarves. Some like to have fun with bright makeup colors or makeup that makes your eyes pop. And yet other women just keep it *au natural.* If you do choose not to cover up, keep in mind that you probably will want a couple hats or scarves just to keep your head warm, since your hair will no longer be helping to keep the heat from leaving your body through your head.

It's also worth mentioning that you will most likely lose hair in other places too: eyebrows, eyelashes, body hair and yes, even "down there." If you shave your legs normally, it's pretty sweet not to worry about them getting stubbly, but it's a little freaky to not have eyebrows or eyelashes. And again, everyone is different, so depending on your treatment and how your body handles it, you may only lose a little hair on the rest of your body, or none at all. You can opt to use some makeup to create eyebrows and lashes, and we suggest getting some help from a professional so that you are comfortable with the outcome.

We told you how crappy losing your hair can be, but you can still make some lemonade out of this lemon—believe it or not. Having a little fun with different wigs, hats and wraps is one way to do it. The other is to realize that there is probably no other time in your life that you will ever be bald. (Um, isn't that a good thing?) What we're saying is that you can use this opportunity to feel a sense of empowerment. Would you have ever dared to shave your head, had you not been losing your hair already? Would you have ever decided to cut your long locks into a cute pixie cut or a spiky "do" if you didn't feel you had to? While it may be frightening to see ourselves without hair, it's also an opportunity to accept and love the shape of your head, not have to worry about blow-drying, curling, or even shampooing your hair! It's kind of liberating. No more bad hair days!

Scary Scars

UNLIKE LOSING YOUR hair, which is usually temporary, some parts of treatment last a lifetime. We're talking about losing body parts, the resulting scars and the scars you may feel emotionally for years to come. If you elect to have some form of surgery as part of your treatment plan, you will most likely end up with a scar or two or lose an organ, some of your feminine parts, a limb or something else. This can be incredibly traumatic—understandably.

Losing a part of your body can feel like losing a loved one, and it's often mourned in the same manner. It can also disrupt your body's equilibrium and may be very difficult to adapt to, physically. It may affect your fertility, mobility, hormones and metabolism. Even if you haven't lost a part of your body, having lasting scars from

Kendall:

When I elected to have a sternotomy to remove the tumor behind my sternum, I was terrified of what the surgical scar would look like. This surgery meant cracking open my chest, just like an open-heart surgery. It would leave a large, seven-inch scar right down the center of my chest. I was devastated and worried about always feeling self-conscious about how low my shirt was or wearing a bathing suit. Everyone would see my ugly scar! But, I slowly began to accept my scar as a battle wound from the Cancer War. Today, even though I don't consider it to be beautiful, I am okay with it and maybe even a little proud to show it, knowing the surgery that created that scar may very well have saved my life. My body may not quite be the same, but then again, neither am I.

surgery can serve as a constant reminder of the cancer crap you've experienced.

You don't have to love your scars or your flat chest or your reconstructed breasts. You don't have to pretend you're happy that you no longer have a thyroid and are taking medication to replace that organ's functions. You don't have to look in the mirror and feel beautiful all the time when you look at those scars. Those scars or new or changed body parts can leave us feeling lost, depressed and just plain ugly. Just like the emotions that stay with us from battling cancer and often haunt us, our physical scars can do the same. It's not easy to accept the crap that cancer can leave with you (or can take away).

However, a huge part of Cancer World is about adapting, accepting and learning to love your changed self, scars and all. Just like the cancer experience itself, our

Lean On Me

Finding support while facing cancer is so important! Friends and family can be wonderful supporters, but sometimes it's best to find a neutral party who isn't personally affected by your cancer status. Check your local community for cancer centers and support groups. Usually your treatment center and local hospitals can provide support information. You may also wish to contact national organizations such as:

- **IMERMANANGELS.ORG**—This group pairs someone facing cancer with someone who has fought and survived the same cancer.
- **211**—Dial "211" on your phone or go to 211.org to locate health and human services, 24/7.
- **IHADCANCER.COM**—A cancer support network that lets you search for people by age, location, cancer type and treatment.
- **WHATNEXT.COM**—Share your cancer journey and connect with others.

scars become a part of us and we can learn to appreciate them, and maybe—*maybe*—love them. Our scars tell a story, and while some chapters in that story are about fear, anger and despair, the rest of the story just might be one of hope, determination and overcoming obstacles.

You might try writing a letter to your scars or missing or changed body parts. It may sound silly, but this exercise can be very healing. You may find that the disgust or sadness you hold for your physical scars is really directed at your entire, tough-as-shit cancer experience. And you just might find that you can learn to love your new body and yourself, scars and all.

Friends Come and Go

JUST LIKE THERE are so many people who truly stick by you through your cancer diagnosis, there are others who may back off or disappear completely. People whom you thought were your friends turn out to not really be the people you thought they were. Just as you may have those golden friends who call, visit you, make you laugh, cook you dinner and help make Cancer World less awful, you will most likely also have the friends who stop calling and basically drop off the face of the earth. Unfortunately, this is all a part of cancer.

If this happens to you, it can be very upsetting. Sometimes the person who vanishes is the one you were sure would be by your side throughout the cancer stuff. We just never know how people will react to someone they know getting a cancer diagnosis. Honestly, for some people it's just too difficult to face. Your girlfriend may be too scared to be able to deal with her feelings—so much that she can't be a friend to you. Or she may feel so uncomfortable and simply not know what to do for you. In that case, it's easier for her to just stay away. Others may just be in denial and are not ready to accept what is happening to you, or they may even have no idea how difficult and how big of a deal it really is. You may even find that as soon as you are feeling better or you've received clear scans, some of those friends who pulled disappearing acts come back. Or, if you continue to be sick and are fighting cancer for a while, or multiple times, even some of the friends who were troopers at the beginning just can't continue to handle it and slowly distance themselves.

Sadly, this disappearing act can also happen with partners, significant others and spouses. Sometimes they just can't hack it. Maybe your husband didn't understand the part of your vows that said "for better or worse, in sickness and in health." Maybe your boyfriend didn't sign up for endless doctor visits and holding your hair back while you pray to the porcelain goddess. Jeesh, what were you thinking when you went and got all sick on them?

Not everyone is cut out to be the supportive friend or spouse for a cancer chick. Does it mean your friend is a bad person? Probably not. A lousy friend? Maybe. Is your man a shitty husband? Well, if he's leaving you because of the cancer, then, yeah, basically. But we all deal with the curveballs life throws at us, or those around us, in different ways. Some people face adversity well and others suck at it. As hurtful and confusing as this can be, we've found that it's better to try to move on and know that your real friends and loved ones—the ones who are able to get past their own issues with cancer—will stand by you. Focus on those positive, shining stars in your life and know that they will be there for you through thick and thin. If you are facing losing a partner or spouse as a result or your cancer status, please find support through those around you or, better yet, seek professional counseling. Cancer is traumatic enough. You shouldn't have to face the other stuff alone.

On the other side of the field, there may be people in your life you decide are not the best to have on your cancer support team. When you are busy kicking cancer you need all the strength, courage and unconditional love you can get. Making the decision to avoid low energy people with negative thoughts might be the best route for you to maintain your spirit during treatment and beyond. There is no need to feel guilty about this. You are fighting for your life and you deserve to have people around you who will surround you with acceptance and the kind of support you need.

New Cancer Peeps on the Block: Previvors

"PREVIVOR" IS A term used to describe those who have an increased risk for developing cancer due to close family history or due to certain genetic mutations (such as mutations of the BRCA1 or BRCA2 genes), but who do not have a cancer diagnosis. In 2007 *Time* magazine chose "previvor" as number three of the top buzzwords of the year, giving millions of people exposure to the term and bringing public attention to the issues that cancer previvors face. According to Facing Our Risk of Cancer Empowered (FORCE), a national nonprofit dedicated to improving the lives of individuals and families affected by hereditary breast and ovarian cancer, the previvor community has its own unique needs and concerns separate from the general population, but different from those already diagnosed with cancer.

If cancer runs in your family, or you are especially young when diagnosed, you may want to consider genetic testing. Genetic testing can help assess your potential risk for cancer and determine if you are a carrier of a genetic mutation that increases the likelihood of cancer development; it does not determine if you have cancer. Those who test positive for one or more of these genetic mutations, our previvor peeps, usually go through a range of emotions upon learning of their predisposition status. Some choose to have prophylactic surgery as a way to prevent cancer, while others choose to get screened more often. Each person must do what feels right for her, from whether or not to test, to how to deal with the results: It is a personal journey with no right and wrong answers.

Genetic testing involves taking a sample of blood, a cheek swab or a tissue sample. It can be complex and so it is important to speak with a specialist in cancer genetics if you are concerned that cancer may run in your family or if you are interested in testing. An expert in cancer genetics can help explain the benefits and limitations of testing and determine whether or not genetic testing is appropriate and likely to give a person further information about his or her cancer risk.

Advice for Non-Cancer Girlfriends

IF YOU'RE READING this and you have not been in Cancer World, but care about someone who is, it's helpful to know how you can be supportive. Cancer can create feelings of unease even with those closest to you, because we often just don't know what to do or how to act. Being open, honest, and just being there to laugh and cry with her is all good stuff. It's okay to ask how the latest doctor appointment or CT scan went. It's okay to ask for clarification if you don't understand the process or what her treatment plan may be. And it's okay to be honest and say you're scared too, but you are here for her.

Even though we've been through the cancer whirlwind, we can't speak for every cancer diva out there. You can't just place a cancer sticker on our foreheads and assume we'll all want or need the same thing. So if you aren't sure what you can do to support your friend or family member, just ask her. Ask her if there is anything you can do for her, and she may very well tell you that she needs to be distracted or she would love it if you made her some dinner (just be sure to find out if there's anything she really wants to eat or anything she can't stomach right now). Maybe she needs a little help tidying up the house or would love it if you could walk the dog while she rests. She might say she's doing really well right now and would love to go for a hike or talk about anything but cancer. Don't be afraid to tell her about your bad day or ask for advice with a situation of your own. There may be times when she can't handle it, but there are also plenty of times when it will feel really good for her to be helpful to you and hear about what's going on in your life.

And don't forget to help her have a life that doesn't focus solely on cancer. Just because she has this crummy diagnosis doesn't mean she doesn't want to go shopping, catch a chick flick or have a night out on the town. It can't hurt to call her up and say, "If you're up for it, I'm picking you up in an hour and we're going out for dinner!" Helping her find activities and events to look forward to and providing a little spontaneity can be fabulous distractions and mood boosters.

Annette:

Once, during a second opinion, the oncologist (several decades my senior) I was interviewing reacted to my concern about losing my hair to chemo with the comment, "Oh, honey, just put on a little lipstick and you'll be fine." Her flip response to my serious concern left me furious. I am sure she never experienced a cancer diagnosis herself, let alone the loss of her hair. How dismissive and superficial her comment was, I thought. And it was. But the concept must have stuck with me in the back of my mind, and I found myself doing small things to help myself look as good as I could while I was going through treatment. And to my surprise, it did help me feel better. Maybe I couldn't wear fancy clothes, but I could get a really nice pair of yoga pants to accommodate my changed body. Maybe I was healing from surgery but I could don a cute front-zip hoodie that felt free and fun. And maybe I was bald, but I could emphasize those beautiful cheekbones I never really realized I had. Sometimes people just say stupid, insensitive stuff. But, on a rare occasion, we can find a sliver of inspiration in there, too.

On the other hand, don't feel like it's your job to make her happy or feel better. It's also not your job to provide a distraction or be the shoulder to cry on all the time. Remember to only do what you are comfortable with. This is a tough time for you, too, and it's important that you talk to other people to help you deal with your feelings around her cancer status.

In the end, remember that she is still basically the same person and she's only human, just like you. She's not contagious, completely fragile or a stranger. Just be yourself, love her for who she is and you will figure out what works best for both of you.

By the way, this advice is just as important while your friend is going through cancer as it is after. Often those around us think that when treatment ends, cancer is over. But it's not that cut-and-dried. Be there for her as she adjusts to her post-cancer-treatment world and comes to terms with the impact this disease has had (and likely continues to have) on her life.

CHAPTER 3

The Healing Power of Real Food

Our society's diet, as a whole, has changed radically in recent times, moving farther and farther away from real food because of modern agricultural practices and food processing techniques. What *is* a real food? Ask yourself several questions. Would your great-grandmother recognize it? In other words, could it come without a bar code? Can you picture it growing in nature? Real foods are those that people have chowed down on across cultures and throughout generations: foods like vegetables and local fruits, whole grains and beans and small quantities of fish, sea vegetables and wild and free-range animals. These are foods that help keep inflammation in check and your body disease-free. Get friendly with them!

FOOD FRIENDS

THESE FOODS ARE like your best friends. They're hard workers and you can always rely on them, whether you are working on preventing or kicking cancer. They decrease cellular damage and inflammation, promote intestinal health and optimal organ function, assist with hormone balance and even help maintain a healthy weight. And don't think that just because they are good for you they taste like crap. Nope! We've got lots of yummy recipes that let these guys shine! Let us introduce you to the Cool Food Crowd. We'll show you why these are the friends you'll always want to have around.

And while we're on the topic, this is the perfect place to mention the importance of getting the health-boosting qualities of these foods into your body through whole foods instead of as a supplement. While supplements can be helpful and can have their place in a healthy diet or during cancer treatment, they are not a substitute for whole, real foods. Your Food Friends are complex creatures. And while some of their star qualities have been brought to light by research and have been isolated into pill form, they likely have many other amazing properties that either haven't yet been pinpointed or gotten as much press. We don't know about you, but your foodie Girlfriends prefer to chew on real chow rather than pop pills, so that's great news to us! Not to mention another important aspect of benefiting from the goodness of foods in the whole, natural state: synergy. Synergy refers to the fact that the health-supporting factors of these foods don't work in isolation but rather in a team kind of approach in which they support and increase each other's superpowers by being consumed together, in a total package deal. This means that if you are swallowing an isolated substance you're probably not getting all the disease-fighting power that you would be if consuming that same substance in a whole food. So use your supplements as needed and directed. But aim to get most of your cancer-kicking power directly from these Food Friends.

Leafy Greens

~~~~~~~~~

MANY OF US are severely lacking in the abundant nutrient supply that comes from vegetables, especially leafy greens, which should be consumed daily. Vegetables, ideally, should make up at least half of your diet. Leafy green veggies, with all of their amazing chlorophyll, nourish your body and provide an uplifting energy. They are superstars in the Cancer-Kicking World! We can't stress enough the importance of adding these amazing plants to your plate. Try eating a leafy green every day for a week and see how you feel . . . and the darker the green the better. Even without changing anything else in your diet, you'll notice a difference.

Dealing with low bone density?

Another reason to eat your greens: They are a fabulous plant source of calcium. This calcium can be absorbed and utilized by the body to build a strong skeleton and prevent osteoporosis. But watch your consumption of spinach, beet greens and chard. These Friends contain oxalic acid, which binds with and reduces the absorbable calcium in these greens (but not in other foods that are consumed at the same time). Cooking breaks down the oxalic acid, and since these greens do contain many other nutritional benefits, don't shun them from your plate completely. A few servings a week is fine; just make sure they aren't your only source for leafy greens. (If you're worried about eating greens because you've been prescribed an anticoagulant, know that you *can* eat them, just be sure to work with your doctor and have your dosage adjusted accordingly.)

Nutritionally, leafy greens are full of fiber, iron, calcium, potassium, magnesium, chlorophyll and vitamins A, C, E and K. They contain high levels of phytochemicals which help prevent and fight cancer, strengthen the immune system, promote the good "bugs" in your intestines, help improve your mood and give you serious energy. Greens are also excellent blood purifiers and support the liver and kidneys. See why you need to get your greens, especially when your body is under serious stress and strain from cancer treatment and from working hard to kick cancer's ass?

Try these leafy greens: kale, spinach, collards, Swiss chard, mustard and dandelion greens, watercress, argula, endive and mesclun greens. (Some of these Friends are also members of the cruciferous vegetable family.) Look for recipes incorporating greens in smoothies, salads, breakfast foods (start getting your "green on" first thing in the morning!) as well as side and main dishes. For those gals working on cancer prevention—as well as cancer chicks in treatment who've checked with their doctor about consuming raw foods—juicing can also be a terrific option for getting more green goodness into your life!

Cruciferous Vegetables

THIS AWESOME GROUP of veggies includes cauliflower, broccoli, kohlrabi, bok choy, Brussels sprouts, cabbage, napa cabbage, daikon radish, rutabaga, turnips and broccoli rabe. Try getting some of these onto your plate every day. Containing powerful cancer-kicking substances such as sulforaphane and indole-3-carbinols, these guys deserve a star role in your diet. They help prevent precancerous cells from becoming malignant tumors and also inhibit the development of blood vessel systems which support tumor growth and survival (angiogenesis).

Annette:

When I was craving comfort food during chemo, nothing made me feel as cozy as warm sweet potatoes out of the oven. Cut them fry-size or in chunks, or bake whole just like a baked potato, and enjoy the sweet, creamy goodness.

If your thoughts around Broccoli & Co. make your stomach want to turn, it may be because you have consumed overcooked, lifeless versions of these veggies in the past. Giving them a short steam or a super-quick dip in boiling water helps preserve their crispness and vibrant green color along with their marvelous array of nutrients and delicious taste. Stir-frying is also a good choice for these veggies, and they can be served solo or with some favorite herbs or seasonings. Another option is to eat them in a different form. Maybe a plateful of cauliflower makes you want to say "blah!" but a creamy cauliflower soup has you feeling all comfy and cared for. Look for some appealing, outside-the-box ways you can add these veggies into your diet.

Carotenoid-rich Vegetables

WHEN YOU ARE adding more and more vegetables to your diet, think colors. Not only does it make your plate look pretty, it gets you more plant cancer-fighting power. Green leafy veggies are high in carotenoids, as are brightly colored fruits and vegetables (think orange, red and yellow). Get friendly with carrots, yams, sweet potatoes, squash, pumpkins, tomatoes (cooked) and beets. These veggies all contain powerful plant substances such as lutein, lycopene and others that inhibit the growth of cancer, support the immune system and help make natural killer cells more effective. Carotenoids act as antioxidants, protecting healthy cells from free radical damage. We are exposed to free radicals from environmental factors such as pollution, as well as a poor diet. They are also created during metabolic processes in the body. When there are large numbers of free radicals in the body, they can contribute to the development of diseases such as cancer. Antioxidants give free radicals the boot before they can attack healthy cells. And when you are looking for a healthy way to satisfy your sweet tooth, try adding some of these sweeter-tasting veggies to your plate. Mmm . . .

Whole Grains

WHOLE GRAINS HAVE been a staple food of the human diet for thousands of years. Grains remain whole when they have not undergone any processing that removes the bran and the germ, those parts of the grain which provide fiber, slowing the digestion of the endosperm (starch) and moderating the release of sugar into the bloodstream.

Refined grains are left with only the starch.

So you don't have to be scared of whole grains just because they're carbohydrates. While it's wise to skip nutrient-poor carbs like refined grains, flours and sugar, whole grains are an excellent source of nutrition, as they contain protein, iron, vitamin E and B vitamins. They are a rich source of complex carbohydrates and provide sustained, high-quality energy. The fiber from whole grains is able to bind to hormones and cholesterol, allowing them to be moved out of the body and leaving the colon squeaky clean.

Getting a variety of plant foods including whole grains in the diet is a sure-fire way to up the number of different phytochemicals available for disease-booting action. "Phyto" means plant—and these plant chemicals, which give plants color, flavor and natural disease resistance are amazing warriors in preventing and fighting cancer in our bodies. Phytochemicals work in tandem with other nutrients in foods, which is why it is preferable to consume them in real, whole foods.

When whole grains are refined, most of the phytochemicals, vitamins, minerals and fiber are removed in the process. What's left is a food that quickly converts to sugar in the body, and this in turn can raise levels of inflammation. Inflammation is associated with chronic disease, including cancer (see the Food Foes section on page 81 for more on inflammation).

There is a lot of misinformation these days surrounding what makes a whole grain a whole grain. Many companies are jumping on the popular, good-for-business whole grain bandwagon, and create the impression that their product is a good source of whole grains. In these cases, what you are usually looking at is a processed food that has been altered and likely does not resemble a whole grain in its natural state. Reading labels becomes a necessity. An easy rule of thumb is that if it doesn't look whole (as in a whole brown-rice kernel) or say it is whole (as in 100 percent whole wheat flour), it's probably not.

Each whole grain serves up a unique taste and nutrient profile, so make sure you mix it up throughout the week. If you have a gluten sensitivity, be cautious of grains and flours such as spelt berries, rye berries, kamut and barley, as well as whole wheat berries. They may not bother you as much as wheat, or at all, but just remember they do contain gluten. Additionally, oats don't contain gluten but can be contaminated by it in grain processing facilities. Brown rice, wild rice, quinoa, amaranth, millet, buckwheat, corn and teff are your best bets for gluten-free grains.

An option for those who do not have a full-blown gluten allergy is trying out sprouted grains. Sprouting activates food enzymes, boosts nutrient content and neutralizes antinutrients like phytic acid, which binds up minerals so your body cannot fully absorb them. These grains can be eaten as whole grains or in baked products made from sprouted grain flours. You can purchase sprouted whole grains and sprouted grain products or you can even make your own at home by soaking your grains for several hours and then storing them in a warm, dark place to encourage sprouting. Also, soaking the grains before cooking aids in digestion, as do additions such as kombu (sea vegetable) and bay leaf while cooking.

Berries and Other Fruit

BLACKBERRIES, BLUEBERRIES, STRAWBERRIES, raspberries and cranberries all contain substances that help eliminate carcinogens from the body, hinder the ability of cancer cells to set up their own blood vessel systems and encourage cancer cells to self-destruct. There are so many ways to get berries into your diet: throw them on oatmeal or into a smoothie, incorporate into fruit salad or add to a green salad. And of course just snacking on berries is a wonderful way to enjoy them, as well. When not in season, frozen berries can replace fresh ones.

It's helpful to add other fruit to your diet in most cases, too. Local, seasonal fruit

Chronic Inflammation

While low levels of inflammation are normal and necessary, chronic high levels of inflammation in the body have been shown to allow the progression of development from precancerous forms to full-blown malignant disease. Food foes such as refined and artificial sugar, processed foods, bad fats and many animal-based foods lead to the conversion of a type of fat—arachidonic acid—into compounds that promote inflammation, which in turn can lead to cellular damage and disease. Food Friends, in contrast, form the basis of an anti-inflammatory diet helping to keep cells healthy and cancer at bay.

is always a good bet (for us that's melons, apples, pears, peaches) as well as more tropical fruits like pineapple and citrus in moderation. If you are going through treatment, you might enjoy fruit best after it has been stewed or baked. Concentrate on consuming your fruits whole so you get all the fiber along with the juicy goodness. There are times or situations when juicing your fresh vegetables and fruit is beneficial, but for the most part, try to get these foods in whole form.

Why are veggies always heralded above fruit in importance in one's diet? Although fruit offers a wealth of phytochemicals, vitamins and minerals (and deliciousness!) it is, in general, not as nutrient-dense as vegetables. So enjoy your fruit, but don't forget your veggies!

Omega-3-rich Foods

OMEGA-3 FATTY ACIDS are polyunsaturated fats and are masters in reducing inflammation. They have also been shown to reduce cancer-cell growth in some types of tumors. The most important of the omega-3 fatty acids are ALA, EPA and DHA. The best sources of ALA or alpha-linolenic acid are flax seeds and flax oil, hemp seeds, chia seeds, walnuts and algae. ALA is also found in some green vegetables, such as kale, spinach and salad greens. ALA is considered an essential fatty acid. Essential means that our body cannot make it on its own and needs to get it from our food. The other two main omega-3 fatty acids are eicosapentaenoic acid (EPA) and docosahexaenoic acid (DHA) and are found in fatty fish (and purified fish oil supplements). If eating a vegetarian diet, the body can convert the ALA found in plant sources into DHA and EPA. These two omega-3s support brain development, healthy vision, heart health and healthy cholesterol levels, as well as boosting mood and helping maintain appetite and a sense of well-being. Whew! Pretty amazing! Just make sure to take a break when awaiting surgery as omega-3s can cause blood to be thinner and should be stopped one to two weeks before any procedure.

Sea Vegetables

SEA VEGETABLES ARE a group of plants that grow in the ocean. You may hear them referred to as seaweed. Sea vegetables have been part of the diet of many native cultures in Asia and the Americas for thousands of years. These awesome veggies contain molecules that slow cancer growth, encourage cancer cell death and protect cells against radiation damage. They also stimulate the immune system, including the powerful natural killer (NK) cells, a type of white blood cell that is essential in rejecting tumors and virally infected cells. Seaweed offers a broad range of minerals including all of the 56 essential and trace minerals so important for our health. It also is a good source of folic acid, iodine, magnesium, calcium and some of the B vitamins. Eating too many processed foods or foods grown in mineral-depleted soil can result in a lack of minerals in the body, leading to cravings for salty or sugary foods. Adding sea vegetables to your diet can help balance your energy levels and alleviate cravings.

The main sea vegetables used in the kitchen are nori (laver), kombu (kelp), wakame (alleria), arame, hijiki, agar-agar and dulse. Sea veggies can be used in soups and salads, to make sushi, shaken onto grains and beans in granulated form, and turned into delicious side dishes. Add a piece of kombu to beans or grains when cooking to up the mineral content and aid in digestibility.

Cancer-Busting Beverages

OFTEN WE DON'T put much thought into our beverages. As long as it is tasty and quenches our thirst, what does it matter what we drink? This approach has led to the situation in which our society gets upwards of 20 percent of its daily caloric intake from beverages. This pumps up not only the calories but levels of sugar and other not-so-healthy ingredients in our bodies. But your beverages can support your health if you chose them wisely. Some smart choices are:

- *Green tea:* Green tea is rich in a type of antioxidant called catechins. This antioxidant scavenges for free radicals that can damage DNA and contribute to cancer, and reduces the growth of new blood vessels required for tumors to grow. It also activates enzymes in the liver that eliminate toxins from the body. Because of green tea's minimal processing, the catechins it contains, especially epigallocatechin-3-gallate (EGCG), are more concentrated. (The decaf process does not impact the catechin levels.) Want to get more green tea in your diet? You can not only drink it, but cook with it as well. Brew extra and use, for example, when cooking soups or grains. Just substitute some green tea for the water. Also be sure to try our Green Tea-Mango Sorbet (306).

- *Pomegranate juice:* Pomegranate juice has powerful antioxidants to help nix free radicals that cause damage to your cells and DNA. This beverage scores high marks on anti-inflammation and has been show to slow the development of some forms of cancer.

- *Red wine:* While it's important to enjoy in moderation (and sometimes not at all, depending on your diagnosis and treatment), red wine does contain a phytonutrient called resveratrol which can slow cancer initiation, promotion and progression. Resveratrol is found in the skin and seeds of the grape and is extracted due to fermentation, making red wine the most concentrated source. It can also be found in grapes (red or purple), cranberries, blueberries and mulberries.

- *Water:* Sure, it's not glamorous and trendy like the latest health drink (and many of those acclaimed "health" drinks aren't so healthy!), but our bodies can't do without water. From staying hydrated to helping to flush toxins from our system, getting enough H2O into your day is important! If you are craving some excitement, you can add a flavorful kick by including a splash of lemon juice or some slices of fresh fruit. Make sure the water you drink is as pure as possible. Filter tap water using a carbon filter or reverse osmosis system, or drink mineral water bottled in glass. For hydration on the run, grab a BPA-free stainless steel bottle and fill and go!

Herbs and Spices

NOT MERELY FOR flavor or as a garnish: Herbs and spices can pack a disease-kicking punch as well.

- *Turmeric:* contains curcumin, a powerful anti-inflammatory compound that can inhibit the growth of cancer cells. When cooking with turmeric, make sure to add black pepper, as it aids the body in the absorption of curcumin. Turmeric is also a component of curry powder.

- *Ginger:* is well known for its anti-inflammatory properties and can decrease nausea from chemotherapy and radiation.

- *Garlic:* protects cells from carcinogens and may disrupt the metabolism of tumor cells. Garlic's close relatives—onions, shallots, leeks and chives—are also members of the *Allium* family and offer similarly high levels of sulfur-containing phytochemicals, which pack a cancer-kicking punch.

- *Rosemary:* stops gene mutations that could lead to cancer.

- *Oregano:* has a very high antioxidant activity and promotes cell death in cancer cells.

- *Parsley:* has the ability to inhibit tumor formation. It can also neutralize carcinogens, such as those from cigarette smoke. It is an excellent source of antioxidants, vitamin C, beta-carotene and folic acid.

Cultured Foods

DID YOU KNOW there are about ten times as many microorganisms in your gut as there are cells in your whole body? Most of these microorganisms are bacteria, certain types of which aid us in everything from digesting our food to supporting our immune system to preventing the over-growth of harmful microorganisms. They are also important in inhibiting the growth of colon cancer cells and in keeping us "regular." Due to the many important roles these bacteria, or "good bugs," play in our gut, it is important to do all we can to keep them healthy and thriving. We assist them by adding foods to our diet that support their troops. These are foods that contain so-called probiotics, sources of beneficial bacteria.

Probiotics have become very popular, and many food companies have created products to market to those looking for an easy way to add some "beneficial bugs" to their diet. However, many of these products, such as sweetened yogurts and probiotic drinks, are highly processed, contain sugar and are not a great choice when looking to support your intestinal health. Instead, you may wish to look for organic, unsweetened yogurt and kefir. (As you'll read later in this chapter, you may even want to limit how often you consume dairy—or not consume it at all—and may prefer to choose nondairy versions of these, like soy or coconut.)

Another excellent choice for adding probiotics to your diet is using naturally

Shout, Shout, Let It All Out

Feeling some serious anger at cancer and life in general? Thinking "This is so freaking unfair!" ? You are not alone! It's natural to be pissed off and bitter. You're dealing with some difficult stuff. The important thing is that you don't hold it in. Talking about it will only help (support groups, counselors, fellow cancer peeps, others). And don't feel you have to hold back—even if a "bad word" doesn't usually cross your lips, sometimes it just helps to say just how much cancer *sucks*! (See, there, we just did it.) There are other times to be prim and proper, but cancer isn't one of them.

Don't want to talk just yet? Try yelling or screaming at the top of your lungs (preferably when no one else is home). We're not kidding! It feels great! Feel like kicking some ass, literally? Get yourself a small punching bag and gloves set up in your home and go for it. Or just punch a pillow on your bed. Do whatever works for you that doesn't put you or anyone else in harm's way . . . just don't keep it all inside!

fermented foods. Fermentation is a simple process used to preserve food. Helpful bacteria (you've probably heard of some of them such as *Lactobacillus acidophilus* and *Lactobacillus bifidus*) proliferate during fermentation and improve a food's enzyme content, increase levels of vitamins B, C and K, deactivate problematic nutrients such as phytic acid, and help to release nutrients from food that would otherwise pass through the intestines undigested.

Vegetables such as cabbage and cucumbers, as well as root vegetables such as carrots and radishes, are some of the most commonly fermented foods, and are typically used as a condiment in a meal. It's easy to make your own fermented food.

Here's how:

First, wash the food and cut it into pieces. Next, place the food you are fermenting into a bowl, add unrefined sea salt, and massage the pieces to release their juice. You can also incorporate herbs or spices for added flavor. Then put your food and its juice into a wide-mouth jar, leaving an inch of space at the top. Seal the jar tightly to prevent air from getting in, as that would interfere with fermentation. Keep the jar at room temperature for two to four days. Later, store the jar in a dark, cool place at about 40 degrees Fahrenheit.

If you are buying fermented food, look for products that are raw rather than pasteurized (unless you are immune-compromised, in which case you may want to be cautious of raw foods; be sure to check with your doctor before consuming). Great fermented Food Friends are tempeh, miso, sauerkraut and kimchee. It is especially important to care for the health of your intestines following treatment with antibiotics or chemotherapy. If you need support beyond food, look for a probiotic supplement with a high count of helpful bacteria to help get your gut back on track.

Nuts and Seeds

NUTS AND SEEDS are nutrition powerhouses! As the embryos from which future plants are formed, they offer protein and a wide array of minerals, as well as vitamins, healthy fats and fiber. They also contain antioxidants that suppress the growth of cancer. Although some people are hesitant to eat nuts because they are high in fat, most of the fat in nuts is beneficial, helping with everything from proper cell function and brain development to lowering LDL (low-density lipoprotein) cholesterol and decreasing the risk of heart disease. Also nothing to sneeze at: Nuts can provide a sense of fullness or satisfaction that actually causes you to eat less of other empty-calorie foods that do nothing for you besides pack on the pounds.

Some of our favorite nuts are almonds, pecans, walnuts, hazelnuts and Brazil nuts (which are an excellent source of selenium, a trace mineral which is anti-cancer). Seed faves are sesame, hemp, flax, chia, sunflower and pumpkin (pepita) seeds. Enjoying these nuts and seeds raw (store in the fridge or freezer), lightly toasted or roasted or in a seed or nut butter (think raw almond butter, not Jif!) are wonderful ways to get their amazing nutrition into your body. There is really no limit to the ways in which you can add nuts and seeds to your diet. From smoothies (throw in a handful of chia seeds) to oatmeal (top with hemp seeds and walnuts) to salads (toss on some pepitas) to side dishes and desserts (top with chopped almonds or pecans), nuts bring health-promoting yumminess to your plate.

Beans, Lentils and Legumes

IN A COUNTRY obsessed with protein, moving to a plant-based, whole foods diet inevitably inspires the question, "Where are you getting your protein?" Be assured that nearly all vegetables, grains, nuts and seeds contain some, and often much, protein. Add beans and legumes to that mix, and you have all the food tools you need to get adequate amounts of protein into your body.

Protein is actually a problem when it plays too large a role in your diet, especially when it comes from an animal. Too much animal protein slows the movement in your intestines (read: constipation), interferes with mineral absorption and weakens the liver and kidneys.

Beans offer terrific plant-based protein and minerals along with a host of other health-boosting benefits. They're a great source of fiber, which is important due to its ability to keep blood-sugar levels stable. This is important because high levels of blood sugar lead to high levels of insulin, a fat-storing hormone, in the body. This creates a drop in blood sugar, or crash. And that leads to cravings, hunger and a cycle of ups and downs that stresses the body, and its ability to produce insulin, raises levels of inflammation (which promotes disease) and also affects your energy, mood and weight. From a cancer perspective, the fiber in beans helps keep your colon clean and keeps toxins moving out of your body. Beans also contain phytochemicals, which inhibit cancer cells and which protect cells from genetic damage that can lead to cancer. These phytochemicals also seem to prevent cancer cells from reproducing, and slow the growth of tumors.

If you fear "tooting" your own horn (if you know what we mean!) with beans, try this: Soak dry beans in water prior to cooking, then once they're in the pot add digestive aids that include kombu, a bay leaf and spices such as fennel.

While nothing tastes as good as home-cooked beans (check out page 257 to learn how easy they are), you can keep canned beans in your pantry for when you are in a pinch. Eden-brand beans are a good choice: They are cooked with kombu and packaged in BPA-free cans (BPA, or bisphenol A, is a chemical that promotes cancer and is found in the lining of metal cans).

One bean that has been a topic of debate in the world of food and cancer is soy. In the past, many doctors were advising those with cancer, especially hormone-dependent cancer, to avoid soy foods, based on conflicting data from animal studies. Recently, however, new research in humans has confirmed what the majority of animal research on the topic of soy had shown: Soy is safe for cancer survivors to eat and may even prevent cancer and cancer recurrence. There is some important fine print to add to the moderate soy consumption (no more than three servings a day) recommendation: It is important that the soy be from whole soy foods, and organic. Organic is important with soy as most soy is now genetically modified (GM) and there are no long-term studies on the effect of GM foods and our bodies.

Eating fermented, or cultured, whole soy foods—such as natto (cultured soybeans), miso (a paste made from cultured soybeans), shoyu (soy sauce or tamari); and tempeh (a pressed cultured soybean cake) is the best way to add soy to your diet. This is the way it has traditionally been used in Asian cultures that enjoy a much lower rate of cancer. Compare that to Western countries where most of our soy is highly processed and genetically engineered and is often modified to create soy protein isolate. The culturing process makes the soy easier to digest, reduces the likelihood of allergies, and allows its nutrients to be assimilated more easily, providing an excellent source of plant-based protein and minerals. Moderate amounts of edamame, tofu, soy milk and soy yogurt appear to be fine as well.

We wouldn't encourage you to eat fake meat with isolated soy protein or take isolated soy phytonutrients like genistein and daidzein. It is always best to eat food in its whole form or as close to it as possible. But it does appear that cultured, organic whole soy foods can be part of the prevention peep's and cancer chick's cancer-kicking diet.

Mushrooms

————～～～～————

MUSHROOMS HAVE BEEN used for thousands of years as both food and medicine, and offer some of the best immune system support on the planet. They are often classified as a vegetable or herb, but they are actually fungi. Mushrooms contribute texture to a dish, and can add their own flavor to food or take on the flavor of other ingredients.

Mushrooms are a great source of B vitamins, potassium and selenium, that awesome antioxidant that protects cells from the damaging effects of free radicals. Shiitake, reishi and maitake mushrooms all contain lentinan, a substance that stimulates the immune system, helps fight infection, and rocks with anti-tumor activity. They can be used to support the immune system during chemotherapy. Even the more common types of mushrooms—white button, crimini and portabella—offer cancer-preventing and -kicking benefits. Add them to soups, stews, stir-fries and sauces.

FOOD FOES

~~~~~~~~~~~~~

THESE ARE THE "friends" who lure us in with their sweet talk and pretty looks but wreak havoc on our bodies. They weaken our immune system, cause inflammation, allow disease to develop and our waistlines to expand. And, unfortunately, they are everywhere. Cut down on the time you spend with them. Or, better yet, don't hang out with them at all. Despite the initial warm fuzzies you may feel, if you take a closer look, you'll realize they don't have your best interests at heart.

Refined and Artificial Sugars

~~~~~~~~~~~~

FROM 1700, WHEN each person was consuming about four pounds of sugar a year, to today, when the average is 180 pounds a year, our sugar consumption has drastically increased over the past centuries. Today it is not difficult to consume more sugar—20 teaspoons—in one sweetened beverage than what our distant hunter-gather ancestors consumed in one year. We all know that our collective waistline has been expanding, and this leads not only to health issues related to obesity and diabetes, but also to cancer.

Cancer loves sugar. It's why doctors use a tool like the PET scan, in which glucose, a type of sugar, is attached to a radioactive medicine. Cancer cells, compared to healthy cells, need larger amounts of glucose to function, and slurp up the glucose in these procedures, then light up thanks to the radioactive marker. These cells are then detected on the scan.

Eating sugar (as well as other highly processed foods) also causes our pancreas to release insulin, to allow the glucose to enter our cells, as well as to release IGF (insulin-like growth factor), which causes cells to grow. So a combination of sugar (cancer-cell food) and IGF (telling cells to grow) is not the combo you are looking for if you want to keep cancer at bay.

What's worse, not only do such habits support cancer growth, according to Dr. David Servan-Schreiber, author of the bestseller *Anticancer: A New Way of Life*, they also boost the cancer cells' ability to invade neighboring tissue. Are you in cancer treatment? Again, according to Servan-Schreiber, researchers have shown in tests with mice with breast cancer cells that those cells are less susceptible to chemotherapy when the mouse's insulin system has been stimulated by sugar.

And of course carrying excess weight around on your body is a risk factor for cancer. Not to mention bouncing back and forth between craving something sugary-sweet and then hearty and salty. Time to stop ping-ponging back and forth between those two extremes, and get more centered and balanced with a diet of plant-based whole foods like beans, grains, fruits and veggies.

Much good can be done simply by dropping all sweetened sodas and sports drinks and staying away from processed food, where sugar is often hidden in large quantities. Become a label reader and be especially wary of high fructose corn syrup, which can cause insulin spikes, fatty liver and leaky gut, and has been shown to contain contaminants such as mercury from its processing. But sugar also hides under ingredients such as dextrose, fructose, fruit juice concentrate and malt syrup, just to name some of the more common ones.

Think artificial sweeteners like Splenda, Equal and Sweet 'n Low are the answer? The jury is out on the link between artificial sweeteners and cancer. Want our opinion? If it has been created in the lab out of ingredients you can't pronounce it is probably not the best thing to be putting into your body! And know that you can't trick your body: Some experts believe that artificial sweeteners can lead to eating more, not fewer calories, as the body craves the carbohydrates it has been "tricked" out of getting by the sweet taste from the artificial sweetener.

What about those times when you do want or need a little sweetness? Try natural sweeteners that have only had minimal processing and keep many of their vitamins and minerals, which we need to be able to metabolize the sugars they contain without robbing those from our own body. Sweeteners we like to use in *small* amounts are brown-rice syrup, pure maple syrup, raw unfiltered honey and unrefined whole cane sugar (sucanat). These should still be used in moderation and as a stepping stone in reducing and even omitting sweeteners in your diet. Or try another solution: Get more sweetness into your life by chowing down on some sweet veggies, like carrots or sweet potatoes or a small piece of dark chocolate. Or add some lusciousness by asking for a hug or doing something loving and sweet for yourself.

Processed Foods

WHEN TALKING ABOUT processed foods, it is good to go back to that question: Would your great-grandmother recognize it? A large part of our supermarkets these days are filled with "food" we cannot easily trace back to a real food source. Many of us eat meals with ingredients made in factories and laboratories rather than by Mother Nature. This large-scale food processing has taken not only much of the nutrition out of the food we eat, it has also separated us from our food—from its source and its preparation—and left us with little plastic trays of frozen food, or bags of convenience foods containing unpronounceable ingredients and devoid of love, care and connection. These foods don't nourish our bodies, nor do they nourish our hearts and minds.

As foods are processed and mass manufactured, importance is placed on keeping them portable, palatable and nonperishable. If this means making them less nutritious for the sake of a longer shelf life or better marketability, so be it. If you are eating foods that are "enriched," know that consuming individual substances can't match getting the complete nutritional shebang found in whole foods.

Not only are important nutrients removed in food processing, but colors, flavors, solvents, preservatives and other substances are also often added to the food we eat. Many of these are known carcinogens at worst and taste-warping at best. When we eat these foods, not only do we put our health at risk, but we also train our taste buds to expect chemicalized, industrial food rather than natural, real food. This is why it can take some time for people who are used to eating these processed foods to adjust to and appreciate the flavor of non-processed, whole foods. Once our taste buds have been "detoxed," however, we can enjoy the delicious flavor of real food as we begin to lose our taste and cravings for these manufactured foods.

Sometimes we don't realize just how much we rely on processed foods until we stop to look. Maybe we start our day with a boxed cereal, then move on to a frozen meal popped in the microwave for lunch, and then end the day with a can of soup and sandwich with lean cold cuts on bagged bread. While all of these products may be labeled as "light," "healthy" and "natural," there's nothing too nutritious about them. If you feed your body this kind of diet, you can't expect to enjoy strong health, sparkly energy and get a great glow. Those qualities come only from the food usually found around the perimeter of the store rather than the inner aisles.

By being connected to real food, by touching and tasting and enjoying it, we are actively supporting our health and well-being in a huge way. Think about what you are putting into your body and how you feel. Does that bag of chips, say, make you feel light and bouncy and nourished? How about that weight-loss shake or dinner that came in a box? Compare that with how you feel when you eat real food, such as a fresh green salad or a warm bowl of vegetable soup. We experienced this ourselves firsthand, and we see time and time again with our clients that leaving

Get Real With
Local and Organic

Certified organic products are, unlike their conventional counterparts, grown without the use of pesticides, herbicides and synthetic fertilizers—nasties that pollute the environment and have been shown to cause cancer. Look for the USDA organic seal as well as local farmers who may not have the seal but operate according to organic standards. In the grocery store, organic produce will be marked with a label code starting with the number 9.

Organic meat, dairy and eggs come from animals that have eaten organic feed, been raised without growth hormones and have not been given antibiotics. And if you're incorporating animal products into your diet, consider the conditions under which the animals are raised. We recommend checking that your meat, dairy and eggs are coming from animals which spent some of their time free-ranging on a pasture and eating the food they were designed to eat (rather than cramped in buildings and cages and fed a diet not native to their species).

A good way to do this is buying local, where you can meet the farmer and see firsthand how your food is being raised. This may seem like a lot to pay attention to, but unfortunately the state of what's on our plate today is much different than even a couple of generations ago when the food supply was not as adulterated as it is now. Use your dollars to support farmers who produce food in a way which is not harmful to the earth, and therefore to us. We want a world in which future generations are not saddled with a cancer burden higher than our own!

the highly processed foods behind and enjoying Mother Nature's chow changes everything completely, from our health to our energy level to how we look and feel.

Especially for those cancer chicks dealing with post-treatment weight gain, ditching the processed crap and shifting to a diet filled with real food will help you get the nutrients you need, as well as shed pounds to reach and maintain a healthy weight. How's that possible? When you eat processed and refined foods, your body, in its innate wisdom, continues to send you messages of hunger, as it searches for the nutrients missing from your diet. This leads to continual grazing, overeating, cravings and a feeling of not being satisfied. Compare that with the feeling after enjoying a nutrient-dense meal from whole foods. Your body sends out signals to shut down hunger, stimulate digestion and create a pleasure sensation in your brain. And achieving a healthy weight by eating food as close to its natural state as possible translates not only into a lowered cancer-recurrence risk, it also makes exercising easier and helps you enjoy life more fully.

Gluten

GLUTEN IS A PROTEIN found in wheat, kamut, spelt, rye and barley. While many people can easily digest this protein, others have a sensitivity and some a full-blown allergy to gluten. How does that happen? In those cases the immune system perceives the gluten as an unknown "invader" and then activates the immune system troops in the intestines. The immune system cells then release chemicals causing inflammation and, in the case of a full-blown allergy, the immune system reaction can destroy the surface of the intestine, causing damage. This damage leads to the inability of the intestines to absorb all the nutrients from the food that one has eaten. Besides these nutrient-absorption issues, gluten can also cause additional immune-system distress. Normally our immune systems are able to take care of mutated cells produced in all of our bodies and which, if not eliminated, could potentially turn into cancer. Peptides in gluten, however, have been found to compromise the immune system in a way that may allow mutated cells to proliferate unchecked, allowing cancer to initiate or spread.

A gluten allergy or sensitivity can pop up anytime throughout life, and can be triggered by pregnancy, viruses, stress or even surgery. Sometimes we might be noticing symptoms in our body and not make the connection to gluten. If you experience issues such as diarrhea, gas, arthritis, depression, chronic fatigue, irritable bowel, bone or joint pain or muscle cramps, you may be showing signs of a gluten sensitivity. Gluten sensitivities are not as few and far between as you might think, so if you are experiencing any of these issues, it is worth taking a closer look.

There is diagnostic testing for gluten allergy (a.k.a. celiac disease) and sensitivity but you can start by simply doing an elimination experiment: Remove all sources of gluten for two to four weeks and see how you feel. (Check out www.celiac.com for a list of "Safe and Forbidden" foods, and read labels to look for gluten-free products.) You may see many or all of your issues disappear or diminish. If you want to check, you can go back to gluten and see what happens. If you start to feel symptoms flaring up again, you have double proof that you're better off going gluten-free.

Worried that you have to miss out on all the food fun if you give up gluten? No need to freak: You can still eat your cake even without gluten! There are pastas, cereals and flours that are gluten-free, as well as lots of whole grains, too—check out rice, buckwheat, amaranth, teff, corn, millet and quinoa. Oats are naturally gluten-free but often get cross-contaminated in processing, so if you want to be 100 percent sure, look for gluten-free oats. Most supermarkets and online food shops now have a dedicated gluten-free section. Just keep in mind that "gluten-free" doesn't necessarily mean healthy. Gluten-free products can still contain other not-so-good ingredients, so be sure to read the label carefully!

Dairy

MOST OF US probably grew up believing grown-ups and ads telling us that milk "does a body good." Following the example of celebrities and the admonitions of our parents, we dutifully emptied our milk cartons at lunch in the school cafeteria and then drank another glass or two at dinner time. Cheese made food delish, and ice cream was our favorite dessert. There was no doubt that dairy was essential to our healthy growth and development, as well as being a symbol for creamy comfort food.

Never mind the fact that no members of other species continue to drink milk after they are weaned. Forget the fact that the cow's milk used to fill those cartons and make that ice cream was meant for baby cows and not humans. Ignore the connection that many dairy-fed kids are constantly snot-nosed, ear-infected and slurping antibiotics.

While dairy has been used (in small amounts, and in a cultured form) in some populations, many of the world's adults do not produce lactase, the enzyme necessary to digest the sugar (lactose) in milk. Eating dairy products then leads to bloating, gas and mucus production, as well as inflammation. As you've learned, inflammation in the body is not the kind of environment you want to support if you'd like to enjoy health and be disease-free. Besides lactose, another problematic component of milk is the protein casein. Some studies have shown that casein may promote cancer development and growth when it makes up a little less than a quarter of the diet. This casein-cancer connection is another reason to leave dairy on the shelf.

Another downside to dairy is hormones. Cows used for milking are regularly given hormones to speed growth and increase milk production. Drinking organic milk, and think you don't have to worry? Even cow's milk produced to meet organic specifications (including milk that is rBGH-free) contains hormones, since dairy herds are

Kendall:

I have to admit I've always been a big cheese eater. In my childhood, even up into college, I loved my grilled cheese sandwiches with the highly processed American cheeses, and Velveeta Mac 'n Cheese. In more recent years I grew to love gourmet cheeses—especially cheddars—and loved to put out a nice platter at get-togethers. If there was cheese in front of me, I would eat it. A *lot* of it. Eventually I made a point of buying organic or locally made cheeses and was happy with that.

So here's the thing: Even as we were writing this book, I realized that I really needed to take my cheese eating down a couple of notches. I know about the whole casein issue and the connection to cancer, so isn't it stupid of me to continue to eat cheese? A lot of it? Yes, I think that's a bad choice for me, personally. Do I still have some every once in a while? Yes, I do. And I don't worry about it. As long as it's organic, local and high-quality.

I've also discovered that I often feel bloated and kind of yucky if I eat more than a couple pieces of cheese on occasion. And it can make me break out with acne. When I avoid it, I don't have those issues.

So luckily, my desire for cheese has greatly diminished. All of the meals and situations in which I normally would be including cheese just don't seem to need it as much. I'm finding other, better alternatives like nutritional yeast, occasionally nondairy cheese, like Daiya, or I just make the dish better in some other way. Cheese is addicting! It's a tough habit to break, but once you do, you can see the light—I promise! There *is* life after cheese.

now—thanks to modern farming practices—kept continually pregnant, and so pass the heightened levels of hormones in their bodies into the milk we drink and dairy products we eat. Ice cream and cheese are concentrated sources of dairy, with ten pounds of milk required to make one pound of cheese.

Not only is the cocktail of hormones in dairy potentially cancer-causing for adults, it is especially risky for our daughters, leading to earlier growth and sexual maturity. The composition of cow's milk is designed to cause significant and rapid growth: from a sixty pound calf to a six-hundred pound cow in about eight months! Why is that bad? Studies have shown that earlier menarche and taller adult height were predictive of an elevated breast-cancer risk.[1]

The most powerful growth-related hormone found in cow's milk, IGF-1 (insulin-like growth-factor-1), has been shown to promote *undesirable* growth as well: cancer. The hormone given to cows to increase milk production, rBGH, or recombinant bovine growth hormone, increases levels of IGF-1.

It is for all of these reasons that we would encourage you to ditch, or at least strongly limit, dairy. Though it may seem like we are suggesting the impossible, we're pretty sure that when you are feeling great and enjoying better health you won't miss it much. There are lots of delicious alternatives for milk: try soy, rice, almond or, our favorite, hemp milk! There are also nondairy cheeses out there but you do have to be a label reader and check: Many of them contain casein.

Another tasty option for replacing cheese is nutritional yeast. Not to be confused with active dry yeast or brewer's yeast, nutritional yeast is a deactivated yeast which has been grown on a molasses-based medium. It is then dried and sold as a powder or flake. The yeast, which is gluten-free, has a cheesy flavor and is rich in amino acids, niacin, folate, zinc, selenium and thiamine, and a great vegan source of vitamin B-12. Check out our recipes for some ideas about how to use this yummy condiment!

For a tropical treat try coconut milk products, including coconut-milk ice cream. Better yet, try our Coconut Ice Kreme with Cherry Swirl on page 303 for some dairy-free goodness!

---

[1] Dr. Catherine Berkey, of Brigham Women's Hospital, in Boston Massachusetts, examined data from participants in the Harvard Nurses' Health Study. Her findings were published in the journal *Cancer* in 1999. Of the 65,000 participants, 2,291 developed breast cancer. Dr. Berkey's comment: "Earlier menarche and taller adult height were predictive of elevated breast carcinoma risk. Our work provided evidence that breast cancer risk is influenced by preadulthood factors, and thus prevention efforts that begin in childhood and adolescence may someday be useful."

Meat

THE TOPIC OF animal protein is emotionally charged for many people on both sides of the "To eat or not to eat meat" discussion. Our family history, eating preferences, view of animals and many other factors come into play when talking about meat. Some of us grew up being told that meat is the best source of protein and as such is essential for our growth and development, making us sure we shouldn't live without it. Others have been surrounded by friends and family who eschewed eating meat for ethical reasons and themselves can't imagine chowing down on anything that had a mother.

There are plenty of not-nutritionally-related reasons for saying no to meat. Caring about our planet, including the animals that inhabit it, and not wishing to do them harm, is a great reason for kicking meat off your plate and a strong motivation for us, personally. For now, for the sake of keeping it on topic, we've decided to stick to talking about meat and the relationship to cancer.

As two chicks who were mostly meat-and-potatoes kind of gals pre-cancer, we know what it's like to believe that eating meat is a no-brainer. Facing a life-threatening disease, however, forced us to consider the merits of a meat-free diet. For us, getting cancer gave us the kick in the pants needed to shape up our diets and our lives so we could support our immune system, enjoy better health and have more energy and radiance than ever before in our adult lives. In terms of diet this meant moving to a plant-based, whole foods diet while reducing, and slowly eliminating, most animal-based foods.

There's plenty of research showing the connection between meat and cancer. But instead of getting all science-y on you, your Girlfriends would like to chat a bit about why we feel that moving meat off your menu, or at least significantly reducing its space on your plate, can mean more health and vitality for your body. Here are some things to consider:

- The fat content of most meat—red as well as white—is troublesome not only from a dietary perspective but also because the fat is where environmental contaminants absorbed by the animals are stored. Since animals are at the top of the food chain, they are a major source of these contaminants, which then burden our bodies and may lead to cancer in humans.

- Nitrites and nitrates, preservatives used in lunch meats, hot dogs and sausages, can be converted to nitrosamines in the body and are known carcinogens. Consumed regularly and over time they can contribute to cancer. These meat products also typically contain many other chemicals since they are made out of the "leftovers" of the meat industry and require other additives to make them palatable and less perishable.

- Meat contains no fiber. Fiber is important for healthy digestion and elimination. A diet low in fiber is a risk factor for cancer, especially colorectal cancer.

- Animals are treated with hormones that are then passed on to us when we eat animal products. These hormones put us at a greater risk for developing cancer.

- We eat much more meat than at any point in human history. The vast majority of meat produced is from animals that are raised in factory farm conditions—not as animals should be raised—and this leads to antibiotic use, species-inappropriate diet (grain-based), and stress and trauma for the animals. These stress hormones are in the meat and we take these into our body when we eat it. And a corn-based diet is not only unhealthy for an animal, it produces meat that is less nutritious.

- Eating more meat usually means eating fewer plants. Eating fewer plants means less fiber, fewer antioxidants, no phytochemicals—all important in preventing cancer.

What is the solution? Answer: moving from a meat-based to a plant-based diet. (Don't panic! You can do this in baby steps.) A plant-based diet has huge cancer-kicking potential as well as providing your body with uplifting, positive energy. If you do eat meat, please consider consuming only organic, grass-fed meat and do so mindfully and in small quantities.

Bad Fats

FATS AND OILS help give us a feeling of fullness and satisfaction. This is why keeping fat intake overly low—as has been the trend recently in fad diets—by filling our plates with "low-fat" foods may lead to overeating and then weight gain. Many low-fat products also use large amounts of sweeteners to make up for the lack of full taste and flavor due to the missing fat. If we eat healthy fats, we are supporting our body, which needs moderate levels of good fats for certain functions like vitamin absorption, brain function, cell-membrane strength, the immune system and cell communication. Here again the rule is the less processed and refined, the better. Oils such as organic cold-pressed extra-virgin olive oil and unrefined organic coconut oil are excellent choices for a cancer-fighting diet. Be sure to store oils in a cool space, protected from light. This protects against rancidity, which turns oils toxic. Also, store oil in glass to avoid hormone-disrupting chemicals found in plastic.

Fats to avoid are refined oils. These are oils that are usually extracted at high heat using a solvent such as hexane. They are then often bleached and chemically treated so that they can hang out on the shelf for a long time and have a neutral color and taste. Even those refined oils that have been expeller-pressed are not as good a choice as unrefined. They have still received further processing and have lost vital nutrients.

Often the temperatures in the refining process are so high that trans-fats are formed. You've probably heard about these health-zapping fake fats that, due to their immune-compromising qualities, are not good choices and can lead to diseases such as cancer. These trans-fats can be found everywhere including in margarine, shortening, processed foods, oil that is repeatedly used in deep-frying, and partially hydrogenated oils.

We've covered a lot of information about our Food Friends and Food Foes in this chapter. Of course much more could be said and there are other books out there that can take those of you who are nutrition geeks, like we are, deeper into the science and research behind what we've touched on here. But our goal in this guide is to get you good, solid information and get you quickly on your way into the kitchen where you can create and enjoy delicious food and support your health. When you focus on the Friends and avoid the Foes you create a diet based on unrefined plant foods which is anti-inflammatory and disease-preventing. Read: cancer-kicking!

CHAPTER 4

Find Your Food Groove

When did food and eating get so darn serious? It's become a mathematical formula, a stress-inducer and a confusing, frustrating maze of what to eat and what not to eat. It doesn't need to be so complicated, and in fact, should be enjoyable, delicious and—dare we say?—fun!

To help you experiment with different foods and food groove options, we've made some recommendations in this chapter. Use them as a guide in exploring what works for your body, without getting too hung up on the details. Even between the two of us, we differ somewhat in our dietary choices and eating habits. And to be honest, that's totally cool. We're all unique and need different things at different times in our lives, and that includes food.

Get Real (Food That Is)

WITHOUT A DOUBT, the most health-promoting type of diet includes real, whole foods, most of which are plant foods, and little to no animal or highly processed and refined foods. It's sad that today we have to clarify by saying "real" food, but we do. There's so much on the grocery store shelves that we call food, which is filled with artificial, chemicalized, processed, refined ingredients that were either stripped of all their real food goodness or never real food to begin with. If you read the list of ingredients on a box of food and you don't know what they are or can't pronounce them—honey, that ain't real food.

Focusing on plant-based foods, especially vegetables and fruit, ups the ante for fighting disease and promoting health. These foods can help to increase energy, balance moods, and improve overall well-being during cancer treatment. They also boost the immune system, lower blood pressure, help to cleanse toxins from your body and assist in maintaining an even blood-sugar level.

The simple version of a plant-based diet which we outline below is a fantastic place to start, especially if you are used to what has become the Standard American Diet (SAD). The SAD diet is what is now prevalent in the United States and includes industrialized, empty-calorie, processed foods and few whole, plant-based foods.

Basic Plant-Based, Whole Foods Diet

- 50 percent vegetables, sea vegetables and fruit
- 25 to 30 percent whole grains
- 20 to 25 percent quality protein (animal, plant or combination)
- Processed foods, refined sugars and red meat in moderation or not at all

HALF OF YOUR diet should include a variety of the veggies we talked about in Chapter 3, paying extra attention to your leafy greens and including some fruit. About one quarter of your diet or meal should contain whole grains like brown rice, quinoa or millet. The last quarter is for protein, which can include animal proteins like eggs, kefir, yogurt, poultry, meat, fish and plant proteins such as beans, legumes, nuts, seeds and cultured soy.

This is a basic guideline for eating that gives you room to discover what works best for you. We like to call this style of eating "flexitarian," because it allows room for flexibility based on your personal needs and circumstances. For example, if you're in the middle of chemotherapy and eating eggs or other animal protein a couple times a week makes you feel stronger, then go ahead! That doesn't mean that having a huge steak (even a grass-fed one) every night of the week is a wise decision, so be smart in your flexibility and pay attention to how your food choices make you feel. (For those going through cancer treatment, there is usually an increased protein need to help rebuild cells. We will talk more about this in Chapter 7.)

By the way, you'll probably notice you don't hear us talking about counting calories or points. Wouldn't that be an amazing way to live—just enjoying your food? You can if you are embracing a plant-based, whole-food diet, a way of eating that makes the need to watch calories superfluous for most people. You'll be eating nutrient-dense, filling foods, so it is unlikely you will overeat (you'll be getting the nutrition you need, so your body won't constantly be on the lookout for more) or feel hungry all the time (real, whole foods are full of fiber and other goodness to help you feel and stay satiated longer).

If it helps, try picturing your dinner plate (or a plate for any meal) divided into the sections below.

Veg Out

-----~~~~~~~~-----

IF YOU'RE READY to kick it up a notch, you can begin to omit meat and fish from your diet as your protein source, creating a vegetarian diet. Incidentally, the proportions remain the same, but the types of protein change so that no meats and fish are included.

In a vegetarian-focused diet, you're still getting plenty of vegetables, fruits and whole grains, but you rely on more plant-based foods as your protein source. This diet requires more beans, nuts, seeds, legumes and fermented soy and can include protein from animal by-products like eggs and possibly yogurt and kefir. Also remember, there is protein in vegetables and whole grains, too. One way to think about the central guideline in a vegetarian diet is no eating anything with legs or a face. Some vegetarians still choose to eat fish and shellfish, which is technically a pescetarian diet. If this approach works for you, then enjoy your seafood occasionally.

Vegetarian eating is very health-promoting and works for most people if done correctly. One of the mistakes often made when trying to maintain a vegetarian diet is the lack of real, whole foods, especially vegetables. If you are a virgin vegetarian, it's a common mistake to knock meats out of your diet, then to focus on eating pastas, breads, some fruits and veggies and getting your protein from pasteurized and processed dairy sources like milk and cheese. This is the wrong way to go vegetarian, which you will soon realize if you pay attention to your body. This type of pseudo-vegetarianism will leave you malnourished, tired, grumpy and probably cause weight gain. Don't fall into this trap!

Vegetarians need to maintain the ratios we discussed above and be sure to get protein from quality sources, like beans, nuts and eggs. Beans are also high in B-complex vitamins and iron, which vegetarians often lack because of the omission of meats. Sea vegetables (seaweed) are also important in a vegetarian diet, because they offer an abundant supply of nutrients that may be more difficult to replace without meat, poultry and fish.

To take it a step further, try a purely plant, a.k.a. vegan, diet. Moving to a purely plant diet is often approached with hesitancy because for some people, it can seem rather extreme and overwhelming. However, if you've already given meat, poultry, fish and seafood the boot, omitting eggs, dairy and other animal-made foods is not a far reach. Again, this diet still follows the same ratios of vegetables, fruit, whole grains and protein, but the protein source changes to eliminate all animal-based foods.

If you are following a strict vegan diet, this means you do not eat anything that comes from an animal or insect—nothing from anything with legs or a face. That means no meats, fish, poultry, dairy, eggs, or honey. Your food comes from plants and only plants.

Why is a purely plant diet beneficial to your health? In Chapter 3 we talked about meat and dairy causing inflammation and increasing the cancer risk. Eating only plant foods can help to prevent and fight a number of diseases including cancer, cardiovascular disease and arthritis, to name a few. Most studies show eggs to be a good source of many nutrients; however, part of the vegan lifestyle is not just about health benefits, but also about the animals used for food and the conditions in which they live. Technically, if you are going vegan, eggs would be omitted for this reason. Fortunately, pastured, organic eggs come from chickens in much better conditions. Having a few eggs per week can be beneficial, providing energy and strength, especially during cancer treatment.

Keep in mind that it is often advisable to take a vitamin D supplement (and get outside in the sunshine!) when on a vegan diet because the diet is missing butter, eggs and oily fish, all of which contain vitamin D. You can also get some vitamin D from mushrooms. B12 is another essential vitamin that a vegan diet is often lacking, so taking a supplement may help. Nutritional yeast—which has a cheese-like flavor—is a reliable source of B12, and can be sprinkled on top of rice, quinoa, veggies and—our favorite—popped corn.

It's often easier to change your diet in steps. Rather than jumping right into a vegan diet when you've been eating meat seven days a week, try working toward a vegetarian diet first. Go for "meatless Mondays" as a starting point, and then pick three days of the week when you will omit meat and add in plant-based protein foods. Focus on adding in the plant-based foods, rather than on what you are taking out.

Another way to experiment with vegetarian and vegan diets is to commit to a weeklong trial run. Be a vegan or vegetarian for a week (although keep in mind that we are just referring to your diet—"being" a vegan or vegetarian also usually incorporates a particular animal-free lifestyle, i.e., no fur coats or leather boots!). Use the recipes in this book to plan out your meals and give them a try for seven days in a row. Whenever you make changes in your diet, it's important to pay attention to how you feel before, during and after eating. Notice if you have more or less energy, better digestion, different moods or clearer thinking. Most likely, if you cut out a significant amount of animal foods from your diet and focus on getting plenty of vegetables, fruit, plant protein sources (beans, legumes, nuts, seeds, fermented soy)

Gratitude

Think we're off our rockers bringing up a topic like gratitude in a book about cancer? Think again! Gratitude is actually a secret, powerful weapon against disease. Yes, it's true! Research shows that those who are grateful have an edge health-wise over their not-so-grateful peers. Grateful chicks are more optimistic and that translates into a boost for the immune system. It also means stress is less of a problem. Want to grow some gratitude? Try our favorite tip and grab yourself a gratitude journal. Pick a pretty one you will enjoy using and place it in a spot where you will see it every day—near your bed or on your desk, for example. Then take a few minutes daily to write down at least ten things you are thankful for. Too hard? Start with two or three then pump your gratitude muscle by increasing that number each week. Need some ideas? Ask yourself what you take for granted in your life. (Do you have a comfortable bed to sleep in? Do you have clean water to drink?) And extend the practice throughout the day by engaging in optimistic, appreciative self-talk.

and whole grains, you will feel an improvement overall, even with specific ailments you may have suffered from previously.

In the Raw

———⌇⌇⌇⌇⌇⌇———

ANOTHER DIET THAT you may have heard about is a raw diet. Just like every other diet, there are different levels of a raw diet. Some raw foodists eat 100 percent raw food. Others eat about 80 percent, while there are those raw foodies who stick to 50 percent. There are big benefits to getting raw foods in your diet, so whether you have a few here and there or jack it up to 80 percent, explore adding in more raw foods and meals.

Eating raw generally means your food is not cooked at all or has not been heated above 118 degrees Fahrenheit. The reason for this is because studies have shown that once your food is heated over 118 degrees, it begins to lose some of its nutrient content. You can eat raw food and *sprouted* raw (living) foods, which we mentioned in Chapter 3. When you eat raw or living food, you're going to get some fabulous uplifting energy. Many people who include more raw food in their diets experience increased energy, weight loss, better digestion, increased mental clarity, improved and more even moods and clearer skin.

To get raw foods in your diet, the simplest first step is to eat raw fruits and veggies. Have an apple as a snack or munch on some carrot sticks. Eat a fresh-greens salad. Try some of the raw food dishes in this book to get started. Once you start adding in more raw foods, you're guaranteed to feel a major increase in energy and moods, so do what you can to get a little raw.

Another way to add raw food to your diet is by juicing. Juicing maintains all the powerful raw nutrients in fruits and vegetables, but removes the fiber so your digestive system gets a break, which allows your energy to be used in other areas of your body. This can help give your immune system a boost too. Juicing also helps to release and cleanse toxins from the body. Just be careful to make sure you are not "fasting" on an all-juice diet, especially for any extended period of time, because you still need to get the fiber the juicing removes on a regular basis.

Try juicing in the morning before breakfast, or even in place of breakfast, followed by regular meals the rest of the day. Juicing is a clean, energizing way to start your day. Juicing is most easily and effectively done with an electric juicer, although it can also be done by mixing fruits and vegetables with a little water in a powerful blender then pouring the blended contents through a strainer to remove the fibrous part.

You will find some juicing recipes in this book, but be sure to experiment and find out what you like. You really can't go wrong: just be sure to stick with mostly vegetables since they have less fructose and won't spike your blood sugar like fruit can, especially with the fiber removed. You can juice cabbage, carrots, beets, broccoli, cucumber, celery, apple, pears, berries, melon, greens, herbs, ginger, garlic, peppers, tomatoes and so much more. Just be sure you don't try juicing a banana—it will just make a big mushy mess. One juicy combination we love is apple, carrot and gingerroot.

A note for immuno-compromised ladies (those undergoing chemotherapy or stem-cell transplants): Be wary of raw foods in your diet, and speak with your health-care provider before consuming raw foods. Raw foods do run the risk of containing bacteria or contaminants that anyone with a weakened immune system may have difficulty fighting off. When these foods are cooked, bacteria are also killed off, so sticking with cooked foods may be a better choice. However, having a few raw veggies or an apple here and there most likely isn't going to cause any harm. Be sure to scrub produce with a brush and even wash with a mild natural soap or specialized produce cleaner. And definitely consult with your health-care provider first.

What's Your Food Groove?

——〰〰〰〰〰——

WE'VE GIVEN YOU some different ways to eat that we think totally rock. Whether you decide to start with the basics and incorporate more plants into your diet, or you want to practice all-out veganism, you are doing some serious good for your beautiful body. We believe, and most other experts agree, that a whole-food, plant-based diet is the way to eat for optimal health. However, you can vary that quite a bit when experimenting with vegan, vegetarian and raw diets and everything in between. Remember the flexitarian approach? Allow yourself room to explore and alter your diet depending on your unique needs and situation.

This is where bio-individuality comes into play. Bio-individuality means that we all have different bodies with unique genetic makeup, blood types, metabolism, genders and ages, so one diet is not going to be perfect for everyone. If we said that everyone should eat a vegan diet all of the time, we'd be wrong. One diet can't possibly be the answer for every body, every day. Needs change from one person to another, based on age, makeup, location, climate, disease, treatment for disease and other changes throughout your life. So don't feel the need to put yourself in a neat little box and label yourself, unless, of course, you want to label your diet and follow it precisely. It's entirely up to you! Just try to eat whole foods, mostly plants and be flexible.

So how do you figure out how *you* should eat? What is the best diet for *you*? Beyond the basic plant-based, whole-foods diet, there is a lot to be interpreted from one person to the next. The answer comes from learning how to listen to what your body is telling you. Sound a little hokey? We're not saying you will suddenly have this out-of-body experience in which a voice will tell you what to eat for breakfast that morning (although we suppose that's possible!). Instead it's learning how to read the subtle signs your body gives you every day and then using those signs to make an informed choice on how to respond to what your body is telling you. Here are some examples of signs your body may give you on a daily basis:

- Bloating and gas
- Constipation or diarrhea
- Stomachache
- Headache
- Other aches and pains
- Acne
- Dry skin
- Psoriasis or eczema
- Fatigue
- Mood swings
- Decrease in energy
- Mental uncertainty or memory loss
- Dizziness

When we have one of these ailments, it's the body's way of trying to tell us that something is off. It's your body asking for something. These aches, pains and discomforts don't just happen for no reason. When your body gives you one of these signs, it's your job to figure out what you need. Bloating and gas may mean you ate something with gluten in it that doesn't agree with your body. Next time try eating gluten-free bread or a gluten-free whole grain like brown rice. A headache might mean you are dehydrated and need to drink some water or that you need to get some sleep. Dry skin, eczema and psoriasis could mean there is a food you are eating that contains something that is not right for your body, like gluten or dairy. Or perhaps you need to add more healthy fats to your diet. Feeling tired? You might not be getting enough protein or the right kind of protein.

So often we run to the doctor or pop a pill, but sometimes that just isn't necessary, and what's really needed is a little (or a lot of) adjusting in your diet. There is certainly a place for conventional medicine, and you should seek medical support if you choose to. However, sometimes we really can figure it out and heal on our own. A big part of that is developing awareness of your body and making that connection between your body and the food you put in it. Some cultures and successful ancient medicine practices believe this is the only way to heal, alongside the use of natural healing remedies.

One way to become more comfortable with paying attention to your body's signs is by keeping a food journal. This can help you keep track of what foods you ate when and what signs your body gave you as a result. Then when you get a headache or you have a day with lots of energy, you will be able to look back at what you ate and consider how it affected you. You may begin to notice patterns with certain foods and this can help you make better decisions the next time you eat. If you find, for example, that every time you eat ice cream or drink a glass of milk you have a stomachache, then you may decide that dairy doesn't sit well with your digestive system, and try to avoid it in the future.

You may also find, as you begin to "upgrade" your diet by adding in more real, whole foods, that you notice positive changes in your body:

- Acne clears
- Skin glows
- Moods are more balanced
- Feel energized
- Aches and pains diminish
- Mental clarity and concentration increase
- Get sick less often
- Digestive issues likes bloating, excess gas, constipation or diarrhea stop or improve

• Rarely have headaches or migraines

• Depression and anxiety lessen or disappear

The following is a template you can use for your food journal:

Day:

Time: Food:

Comments *30 to 60 minutes after (physical, emotional, mental)*_____

_____

Comments *2 hours after (physical, emotional, mental)*_____

_____

Making changes in your diet can often feel overwhelming, so it's important to take it one step at a time. Of course, if you have a diagnosis, you will first want to discuss the details of your particular cancer with your physician, since your cancer-treatment protocol may affect what you can or should eat. Once you are clear on that, finding support and guidance from the right people can make all the difference in being successful or not. Health coaches, naturopathic doctors and other professionals who understand the link between food, the body and disease and who treat the whole person and root of the problem, and not just the symptoms, can offer that support. Just be sure you are comfortable with the professional you choose to work with and that your beliefs jive with his or hers. Make sure this person listens to you, addresses your concerns and helps you with a plan of action and doesn't simply throw suggestions at you without any follow-up or support in implementing that plan.

And a piece of advice: Don't think you have ever "slipped up" too badly or too long nutritionally, and that you might as well just give up. Life's not about how many times you fall out of the saddle, it's about how persistent you are at getting back up in it again. And sometimes again. And again.

Water Yourself

Throughout this book we talk about the importance of water and hydration, but how much water do we really need? The answer varies from person to person and at different times or in different situations in your life. For example, when you are enduring cancer treatment, you will need to up your water intake. If you are very active, pregnant or breast-feeding, or if you are in an especially hot climate, you will also need to drink more water. A general rule of thumb, however, is to drink half your body weight in ounces. So if you weigh 160 pounds, you will want to drink approximately 80 ounces of water in a day. And just remember that if you're thirsty you're already dehydrated! Don't let yourself get to that point!

You Are What You Eat

NO MATTER WHAT your food groove is, it's important to remember that your mind, body and spirit are literally shaped and influenced by what you put into your body. Make sure that your food is what you want to be making into *you*! Do you want to have the insides (and outside) of someone who eats greasy chips, pizza and soda all day long, or the person who consumes a variety of brightly colored veggies, whole grains, plant proteins and water?

When you take a bite of food, what happens? You chew it, it works its way down to your stomach where it is broken down and eventually makes its way to your intestines, where it is absorbed into your bloodstream. And where does your blood go? Everywhere! That food enters every cell in your body and is carried into your muscles, tissues, bones, organs, skin, hair, teeth and nails. It even becomes your

Let's Get This Party Started

There's nothing like getting slapped with a cancer diagnosis to make you realize how short life is. How often are we running here, there and everywhere, forgetting to take the time to celebrate and enjoy life as we go? Ironically, it was getting cancer that, for some of us, caused us to really wake up to our lives, moment by moment, and to make the decision to enjoy each day for all it was worth. This celebration of life can take place in big and small ways: from dancing in the kitchen, to singing along to your favorite music at the top of your lungs in the car, to throwing a party "just because." Whatever you do, whatever it is, celebrate the moment. Celebrate your life.

thoughts and emotions! You truly are what you eat.

Realizing you are what you eat means becoming interested in and curious about what lands on your plate, because it will become part of you. Not only does this apply to the actual foods you are eating, but also the quality of that food. Is it fresh or old? Is your produce organic or sprayed with chemical pesticides? Is your meat from an animal that lived a quality life in healthy, natural conditions, or one raised on an unsanitary factory farm? Not only do the nutrients in these foods enter your body, but the characteristics of these foods become you. Food from stressed, sick animals brings that energy into you. Old, wilted veggies contain old, wilted energy.

So when you are choosing your food try to pay attention to the quality, where it came from as well as what it is. Do you want to feel and look vibrant, healthy and strong? Eat nutrient-dense foods that will help you accomplish that: clean, fresh, whole foods, plant-based, and little to no processed foods, refined sweeteners and poor-quality animal foods.

Have Fun in the Kitchen

~~~~~~~~~~~~

NOW THAT YOU'RE familiar with some healthy, simple types of eating, it's time to let loose and have a little fun in the kitchen! For some of our girlfriends, the idea of putting fun and kitchen in the same sentence would never enter their pretty heads. Time to shake up that notion. Getting in the kitchen can be a blast! It's one of the things that all of our health coaching clients report back to us: "I never realized how fun and creative cooking can be!" There's something about chopping fresh veggies, appreciating the colors of the fruit going into the salad, pulling warm sweet potatoes out of the oven and chowing down on good, real, nourishing food, that puts a glimmer in your eye and actually has you looking forward to hanging out in the kitchen. Bring on the fun, pleasure and enjoyment!

Here are a few things we love to do to make our kitchen experience a little more fun. Wear a pretty ruffly apron. Put on your favorite tunes and dance around a little. Make yourself a Citrus Spritzer (page 317) to sip while you cook. Invite a couple of friends over and have a tasting party where each gal creates her own dish. Get your kids involved. Cook with your spouse or significant other.

For those of you going through cancer treatment, round up your family or your girlfriends for a cooking extravaganza. If you are feeling too pooped to chop, pull up a chair, sit back and relax while drinking Sweet Ginger Tea (page 314), and take in the love of those cooking for you.

Try out some new recipes and have your gal pals whip up some food for you (and some for them to take home, too). Feel great knowing that you are doing something that is not only fun but also supporting your body. Once you've experienced the power of real food, and can taste the love that you put into it, the kitchen becomes your sanctuary, your pharmacy and your playground.

CHAPTER 5

Take It One Step
at a Time

When experimenting with new foods and transitioning to a healthier diet, it can sometimes feel overwhelming if you are trying to make too many changes at once. And if you're in the midst of the cancer fight, you may feel ridiculous pressure to go to extremes and make rapid changes. However, accelerating from zero to sixty in a day is a lot, and probably not the best way to change your eating habits. Instead, add in new whole foods in baby steps and take it one step at a time.

If you've been consuming four cups of coffee and two donuts for breakfast most days of the week, and the idea of suddenly sautéing bok choy, kale, daikon radish and tofu and chasing it with a ginger-carrot-beet juice sounds far too daunting, well, take it down a notch. Try two cups of organic coffee, add a glass of water and go for a whole-grain bagel and some fresh fruit. The point is there are different levels and steps to improving your food groove, and we are here to help you figure it out.

We also want to mention that when you are in the middle of treatment and facing all the cancer ickyness, sometimes you may just want to eat a boxed mac 'n cheese and forgo the salad and brown rice. And that's okay. We know, and now you know, that is not a very healthy choice. But if that's all you can handle making and eating once in a while, don't worry about it. At least get the organic mac 'n cheese. You can get your kale in the next day or at the next meal.

Taking steps to improve your diet also means you will have setbacks and times when you "fall off the wagon." Remember, you aren't on a strict diet; you're just working on making improvements as you are able and doing it in baby steps.

Sometimes you can do more, sometimes you can't. Realize that you're only human, and that change takes time. On the other hand, change also takes determination and commitment, so there can be a delicate balance in making choices about what goes on your plate.

The other interesting (and amazing!) part of making these types of positive changes in your diet is that your tastes begin to change and then continue to do so. As you add in healthier, whole foods, your body begins to prefer them more and more. That also means it wants less and less of the not-so-good stuff, like highly processed foods, lots of animal foods and sweets. And this can happen pretty quickly! Your body actually changes its cravings on a cellular level, and this is felt when you realize you no longer care all that much about having that poor-choice food, like that cookie. You feel balanced and energized from all the good stuff you've

Work It, Work It!

Don't let cancer turn you into a couch potato. Sure, you'll have days, especially if you're going through treatment, where you just don't have the energy or you feel plain sick. But, getting some movement into your day doesn't have to mean running six miles. Just going for a ten-minute walk can help on days when you feel beat. On better days, go for a hike, ride your bike, walk a few miles or run. Ask a friend or family member to join you. And if you were a very active person before, there's no reason you can't maintain your level of activity for the most part. Just listen to your body and don't overdo it. The point is, the more you move, the better you will feel and the stronger your body will be in fighting cancer or anything else that comes its way. And exercise releases endorphins, which make you feel happy!

been eating, and the cookie just isn't as appealing. Your body is saying, "Amen, sister! I'm finally getting what I need, and it feels awesome!" And you agree. Believe us—this really does happen!

When you focus on adding foods in, instead of creating restrictions on the foods you shouldn't have, it's much easier to make changes that stick. That's exactly how we transitioned. We set our sights on cool, new, nourishing whole foods, more veggies and interesting new recipes, and had fun doing it. We didn't restrict or count calories, make lists of forbidden foods or scold ourselves if we ate something "naughty." We just kept eating the good stuff and noticed how our tastes and preferences in food changed and our cravings seemed to fade. Pretty cool!

Poor, Better and Best Food Picks

MAKING CHANGES IN your diet in small steps often works well because you can add in new foods little by little and reduce not-so-good foods little by little. This helps to keep it from becoming too overwhelming. Even so, it can be helpful to have some guidance in making decisions around food. Maybe you know a donut is bad news, but what about the whole grain bagel—is that an okay choice or an excellent choice? What would be even better? This section will help you in determining which foods are not so great choices, and which are pretty good or great!

Flours and Flour-Based Foods

POOR PICK: *White Stuff (white flour, white-flour bagels, breads, pastas with added sugar and undecipherable ingredients that you can't even pronounce).* These are everywhere and do your body far more harm than good! These foods contain mostly empty calories, so they fill you up without providing essential nutrients, and then you often feel hungry again sooner. These refined-flour products clog up your body and promote inflammation. If you've got the white stuff going on, try to boost yourself up to the next level.

BETTER PICK: *Processed and Mostly Unrefined Whole Wheat and Whole Grain (whole-wheat and -grain flours, whole-wheat and -grain bagels, breads and pastas).* Whole-wheat products are becoming the popular healthy choice, and are indeed a big step above your white-flour food imitators. Check those ingredients and if it has "whole wheat" it's closer to the whole-grain food that nature actually produced. If it just says "wheat," forget it. That's really no better than the white stuff. You can also find pastas, breads, bagels and crackers made from brown rice, quinoa and spelt. These are fantastic choices!

BEST PICK: *Whole Grains (brown rice, wheat berries, quinoa (keen-WAH), oat groats, millet and spelt).* In their whole form, these are by far the most health-boosting choices. Take it a step further and try sticking with gluten-free whole grains, since gluten can cause inflammation in our bodies, which can lead to disease (remember reading about this in Chapter 3?) Quinoa, brown rice, millet and buckwheat are good gluten-free choices. Never even heard of some of these, much less cooked them? Don't worry; we've got the recipes to show you how. Give them a try and get cozy with whole grains—they should be a staple in most diets.

Sugar and Sweeteners

POOR PICK: *Refined Sugars (white sugar, brown sugar, high-fructose corn syrup) and Artificial Sweeteners.* These are sweeteners that have been greatly processed and refined, leaving little to no nutritional value. They can easily spike your blood sugar and wreak havoc in your body. Aspartame (AminoSweet, NutraSweet and Equal), saccharine (Sweet'N Low), sucralose (Splenda) are some of the artificial sweeteners often found in processed foods and beverages. Be very wary of these and stay as far away as possible.

BETTER PICK: *"Natural" Sweeteners (raw unfiltered honey, pure maple syrup, sucanat, unrefined whole-cane sugar, molasses, raw agave nectar, brown rice syrup and stevia—in green or brown, not white).* Much better options when using sweeteners in baking, your morning cup of coffee or as an ingredient in processed foods. These tend to be gentler on your body, are generally less processed and refined and won't spike your blood as much as highly refined sugars. This can vary, however, depending on the quality, brand and other factors. Use these as a stepping stone to reducing and hopefully omitting sweeteners in your diet. Any sweetener in your diet is too much—use them sparingly, if at all.

BEST PICK: *Naturally Sweet Food (fruit such as dates and date sugar, bananas, apples and figs, and sweet vegetables such as carrots, beets, sweet potatoes, onions and squash).* These are foods worth including in your diet for a number of reasons,

Just Say No to GMOs

We strongly recommend avoiding food that is genetically modified. There is a lack of verifiable studies showing the safety of genetically modified organisms (GMOs) and scientists warn that GMOs may increase cancer risks, along with other uncool things like harming plant and animal species, producing antibiotic resistant pathogens, increasing the use of toxic pesticides and the like. The problem: GMOs are everywhere. Need some help? Check out the Non-GMO shopping guide (smart phone app available) at NonGMOShoppingGuide.com for the lowdown on ingredients to avoid and companies that pledge not to use GMO ingredients. You can also look for packaging labels which state that a product is GMO-free, and can also buy organic. Certified organic products cannot knowingly include any GMO ingredients.

one being that they help curb that sweet tooth. Adding more of these foods into your diet can help to crowd out the less healthy sweets mentioned above. Using dates (and date sugar, which is just ground-up dates), figs, beets, applesauce or bananas in baking is a fantastic way to use fewer sweeteners. Be sure to check out our recipes for some easy ways to add in these foods.

Animal and Plant Protein

POOR PICK: *Large amounts of animal protein from poor-quality sources (beef, poultry, dairy and seafood).* These have been shown to adversely affect your health. These foods have even been specifically linked to higher cancer rates and more inflammation in the body. Even worse, eating a lot (or any) animal protein from an unknown source means it's likely from a factory farm. Not only is this an unspeakable life for the animals, but it also becomes a part of your body when you eat the foods that result from it.

BETTER PICK: *Smaller amounts of animal protein, from organic, humane farms; no dairy, adding in more plant protein.* Consuming meat or other animal protein from animals raised humanely and without hormones or antibiotics, in small amounts, occasionally, is a better choice. Look for organic labels and, better yet, find out about the farm's practices. Stick with local, and get to know your farmer. Also, cut dairy out to avoid the casein (we talked about that in Chapter 3, too). Begin adding some plant-protein foods (beans, nuts, seeds) to your diet as well.

BEST PICK: *Plant Protein (nuts, seeds, beans, lentils, legumes and cultured soy), pastured, eggs and small amounts of quality animal protein, or none at all.* These are the best sources of protein. Don't forget that whole grains and vegetables also contain protein. Eating these protein-rich foods in lieu of animal protein will most likely make you feel fabulous and energized, and will help to fight growing cancer cells. Add these foods in where you can—snack on almonds, cook up some beans to go with your rice and veggies and enjoy cultured soy in recipes like Marvelous Miso Soup (page 279).

Fruit and Vegetables

POOR PICK: *Little to no fruit or vegetables, or canned or frozen in sauces or sugar.* It's clear that we need fruit and veggies in our diets, so the worst thing you can do is just not eat them at all. Even getting some spinach and onion on your pizza is better than nothing. Watch out for packets of vegetables that come in their own sauces or butter or fruit drenched in syrup (for example, those little fruit cups).

BETTER PICK: *Non-organic canned or frozen items without sauces or added sugar, or "fresh" produce from a grocery store chain.* It's much better to get your fruit and veggies from these sources than not at all. Even though grocery stores don't usually carry the freshest produce (which means they've lost more nutrients), they're still good for you, so eat up! Even eating non-organic vegetables and fruits that have been sprayed with pesticides during the growing season is better than not eating any.

BEST PICK: *Fresh, locally grown, organic produce.* By far, the best way to get your fruit and veggies is from a local farm or farmer's market where the food is fresh and preferably organic or very minimally sprayed. Plus, there's something so enjoyable about going to a market or farm stand, picking out the fresh produce and knowing that it came from a clean family farm in your community. It connects us to nature and makes us feel good about the food we are eating.

Beverages

POOR PICK: *Drinks with lots of ingredients, including sugar and artificial sweeteners and dyes like red dye 40 and yellow 5.* Stay far away from these types of drinks. Many "diet" soft drinks, iced teas and sports drinks contain these types of ingredients, and we are often tricked into thinking they are good choices because they say "fat free," "zero calorie" or "energy drink." Read the ingredient label, and you will see that most of these have ingredients that aren't even a food (or a beverage)!

BETTER PICK: *All-natural soft drinks and juices with no added sugar.* It's becoming easier to find all-natural and organic soft drinks that contain little to no sugar or a less refined sweetener, like honey. Getting 100 percent juice is far better than drinking a fruit punch.

BEST PICK: *Filtered water, coconut water, herbal teas.* It all comes back to water: Our bodies can't survive without it, so drinking plain old water is key. Try adding sliced lemon or orange if you like a little more flavor. Coconut water is an all-natural source of electrolytes and is a much better choice than the sport and energy drinks on the shelves. Herbal teas can help heal and strengthen our bodies, and there are many kinds to choose from.

Agricultural Practices

POOR PICK: *Factory farming; conventional practices using chemical pesticides, fungicides and fertilizers; genetic modification.* Factory-farmed animals live in unsanitary, inhumane conditions and are given food that is not only unnatural for their species to consume, but sometimes not even real food at all. These animals are also usually given antibiotics to counteract these disease-ridden conditions. Much of the meat that is available in grocery stores, unfortunately, is in this category, and we highly recommend avoiding it at all costs. This is not "food" you want to put into your body. In addition, conventional produce is sprayed with pesticides and fungicides to keep pests and fungi away. Those chemicals go into your food and accumulate in your body over time, contributing to inflammation and disease.

BETTER PICK: *Smaller farmed food; limited pesticide and fungicide application.* A better choice is to get your food from smaller farms, even if they don't have all-natural organic status. Many small farms incorporate more humane, natural practices than those in the poor-picks category. Some may apply only a small amount of chemical pesticide, fungicide or fertilizer, or spray only once during a season. These choices are far better than the poor picks, but we highly recommend getting your food from the "best picks" section whenever you can.

BEST PICK: *Small local farms; fresh; organic (certified and non-certified); grass-fed; pastured, free-range; know your farmer; grow your own.* The best choice for your health is to eat food that is grown or raised in clean, natural conditions, native to the species and without the use of chemicals, hormones or antibiotics. Often this includes food that is certified organic, although many small farms have organic practices but haven't gone through the certification process, or simply can't afford the expense. Sometimes even "organic" isn't the best choice, depending on the farm: Animals that live in cleaner conditions and meet USDA certification standards, may often still be receiving feed that is not natural to them, such as grains, rather than being allowed to roam free all day to eat grass. This is because the USDA standards do not require these conditions. Even produce that is grown on USDA certified organic farms may sometimes receive treatments to preserve freshness or hasten ripening on the way to the store. We say get to know your farmer and buy directly from him or her if at all possible. Visit the farm—find out how animals are raised and how produce is grown and make sure it is suitable for clean, natural eating. Or try growing some of your own food—from a few potted plants to a large vegetable garden. You can't get food that's any more local or fresh than that!

Methods for Cooking Your Food

POOR PICK: *Microwaving, grilling, broiling, deep-frying or overcooking food.* Microwaving your food may pose some health risks. First, when you microwave your meals in plastic or paper containers, carcinogenic toxins can leach out into your food. These chemicals may include polyethylene terpthalate (PET), bisphenol A (BPA), toluene, benzene and xylene. Microwaving fatty foods in plastic containers can also leach known carcinogens, called dioxins, into your food. On top of that, cooking your food in a microwave oven changes the chemical and molecular structure of the food, which may have damaging effects on your body. It also reduces the nutrient content of the food. Microwaving may be convenient, but it's really quite easy to heat up your food in a pan on the stove with a little water or oil. Try it and you'll see!

Grilling food also creates some potential health problems. The grill smoke contains polycyclic aromatic hydrocarbons, which are cancer-causing chemicals. Additionally, heterocyclic amines form when food is cooked at a high temperature, such as those used in grilling and broiling. These chemicals have also been linked to cancer. Advanced glycation end-products (AGEs) are also formed when meats are cooked at high temperatures. Research has shown that AGEs accumulate in your body over time and can create inflammation and increased risk of kidney disease, heart disease and diabetes. So if you love to grill in the summertime, keep the temperature low and stick to grilling veggies!

BEST PICK: *Steaming, water sautéing, pressure cooking, baking, poaching, cooking on a range or stove top, eating raw food (no cooking).* Steaming your food (but not for too long) and sautéing foods in a small amount of water are ideal cooking methods because they retain many of the nutrients. Other cooking methods, like boiling, are also better choices—just be sure not to overcook. Using your oven and stove top are much better choices than using your microwave or grill. And sometimes just eating your food raw is the best choice!

Cookware

POOR PICK: *Teflon; nonstick.* Studies have shown that perfluorooctanoic acid (PFOA), a toxic, synthetic chemical used in the manufacturing of nonstick coatings in cookware, can be lethal to birds as it is heated and gassed off into the air from the nonstick coating. DuPont, the maker of Teflon (which is the polytetrafluorethylene or PTFE coating itself) offers a brochure advising not to use their cookware near birds for that reason. If it is lethal to birds, it also isn't safe for humans. Other studies show that the coating when scratched and flaked off into food poses little risk to humans; however any synthetic material that might get into your food is best not consumed. While non-stick cookware may make cleanup extra easy, it just isn't worth the risk.

BETTER PICK: *Aluminum, stainless steel, copper lined with stainless steel.* Aluminum is a much better choice than nonstick cookware, although trace amounts of aluminum can enter food and be absorbed by the body. This is more apt to occur if cookware is scratched and dinged, and especially when cooking more acidic foods like tomatoes, fruits or anything with vinegar. Stainless steel may also leach trace amounts of metals, such as aluminum, titanium, nickel and carbon steel. Experts disagree on just how much of a risk, if any, this poses to our health.

BEST PICK: *Cast iron, ceramic, glass, metal with ceramic coating.* Cast iron leaches iron into food, and that's a good thing! Hey, if you're anemic from chemotherapy or for any other reason, getting that extra iron is a bonus. Cast iron needs to be cleaned with water only (no soap, unless you want your food tasting like it) and, once dry, seasoned with an oil such as olive or grape seed. This just means taking a cloth or paper towel and rubbing the inside of the cookware with a small amount of the oil. It's easy! Another benefit to cast iron is that it retains heat once the heating element is turned off, so it saves energy.

Glass and ceramic cookware are also great choices, and don't leach anything into your food as long there is no chipping or scratching. It's also important to purchase this cookware from a reputable source and in the U.S., so that the cookware is likely to meet regulations making it safe from components used in making them, such as cadmium, lead and pigments.

Setting Goals

ONE OF THE suggestions we often make is to create small goals—two or three—that you can work toward each week, month or as frequently as you'd like. If, for example, you are trying to eat more leafy green vegetables but the thought of preparing them every day for a week sounds like too much, make your goal to eat leafy greens on three or four days for a week or two. Then increase it to five. Perhaps your goal is to plan out dinner for five days of the week so you aren't left without an answer to the "what's for dinner?" question. Or maybe you'd like to focus on breakfast and plan to make a power-packed smoothie and some steel-cut oats for a week or two.

The point is, don't make yourself feel like you need to completely overhaul your diet in just a single week. It's often best to take it in baby steps, and you'll probably find that the changes you make will become permanent habits, rather than short-term solutions. Remember, this isn't a three-week diet: It's a new way of life!

To get started check out our sample weekly goals below. Keep in mind these steps are simply guidelines that are not personalized to your comfort level, schedule or preferences, and you may wish to modify or take different steps altogether. Do what works best for you and have fun with it! No matter how big or small the steps are that you take, you're making significant changes in your health, and your body, mind and heart will thank you for it.

Week 1—Focus on Leafy Greens and Breakfast
• Choose one or two leafy greens to try, and eat on three to seven days.
• Eat a healthier breakfast (try a smoothie or steel-cut oats) for three to seven days.

Week 2—Focus on Whole Grains and Quality of Food

• Choose one or two whole grains, like brown rice or quinoa, and add in for three to five days at lunch or dinner.

• On your next grocery-shopping trip, try shopping at a local health-food store (if available) and substitute organic and local options for at least five food items. Start reading ingredient lists on labels, looking for whole foods.

Week 3—Focus on Protein and Hydration

• Try eating only plant-based proteins and no animal foods for one to five days of the week.

• Start the day by drinking 16 ounces of water and drink a total (in ounces) of your body weight divided by two. (Example: for a 150-pound person, 150 divided by 2 is 75 ounces of water.) Purchase and try coconut water after exercise, chemotherapy or surgery.

Making Cents

~~~~~~~~~~~~~~~~

"HOLD ON THERE, Girlfriends!" you might be thinking, *"how am I supposed to upgrade my diet without going broke?!"* Fair question! We're here to let you know that keeping your body and your bank account healthy need not be mutually exclusive. But remember, you do have to be willing to make healthy eating and living a priority, which includes not only investing time and effort but also financial resources. If you are going to increase your budget or spending in any area of your life, food is a top choice. When you invest in clean, quality food, you're investing in your health. Without good health, life is a tough road. Your investment will, however, pay itself off many times over in terms of health, well-being and saved visits (and payments!) to the doctor's office. So, don't be afraid to wisely splurge a little when it comes to your food.

We do use some cool superfoods in our recipes and encourage you to try them, but they can be pricier than your basic whole foods. Fortunately you don't need to break the bank to eat clean, whole foods. Below we've outlined some ways to keep the cost down when eating a healthy, plant-based diet.

Here's some advice for getting the best nutritional bang for your buck:

• Buy whole foods and skip processed, boxed, packaged foods.

• Purchase nutritionally dense foods, and avoid those that don't offer much nutritional value.

• Eat grains, beans and legumes rather than expensive animal products.

• Buy in bulk and skip individually packaged items.

• Look for sales on items.

A Note for Partners and Spouses (and Other Caregivers)

Sometimes the hardest thing for your cancer-fighting gal to do is to think about what to eat next. Trying to plan out meals and then actually create them can be a lot at times. Helping her with this task can offer her a much-needed break. Aren't sure what to cook? Try out the recipes in this book—just remember that sometimes it does take some planning ahead. Pick a few recipes, make your shopping list based on those ingredients and head to the grocery or health-food store. Then you'll be ready to make your sweetie a tasty and healthy meal, which she will truly appreciate. It would also be wise to ask her if there's anything she doesn't feel she can stomach, or any food she'd really like to eat, because sometimes those cancer-confused appetites can be finicky. And lastly, know that your support in the kitchen (even if you aren't totally comfortable cooking these new foods) is a huge relief, especially on those days when she's just pooped.

- Keep it simple: stick with basic veggies, whole grains, beans and legumes.

- Buy dried beans and cook them, instead of canned (page 257).

- Make your own granola instead of purchasing it (page 214).

- Make your own vegetable stock instead of purchasing it (page 271).

- Cook at home rather than buying meals and snacks out.

- Grow some of your own food. Start small with two or three plants in a window or on a balcony, or grow your own garden outdoors.

- Join a CSA (Community Supported Agriculture) or co-op.

- Make larger batches of recipes, then freeze or refrigerate and eat for a few days.

- Avoid impulse buying: Plan your meals before you shop, take a list and don't go to the store hungry.

- Drink filtered tap water rather than buying specialty drinks.

- Look for store brands and stock up during sales.

- Buy in season and local.

- Blanch and freeze veggies from your garden.

- Learn how to can and preserve food from your own garden or from the farmers' market.

Meeting Resistance

IT CAN BE hard enough to make our own changes in life and find a way to adapt. It's even more difficult when family or friends aren't supportive and show resistance. Trying to eat healthier foods that may be foreign to those around you may drum up a few interesting comments: "What are you eating—bird food? Where's the cheese-burger?" Don't let this faze you. You're doing something wonderful and important for your body, and that should feel good physically and emotionally.

A little trick we'll share with you is to play the cancer card if you need to. If someone feels the need to comment on your cuisine—"Oh, you're eating that healthy stuff"—let them know that yes, you are, because you want to eat the best food that will help you fight the cancer. That will shut them up pretty quickly.

Another thing to keep in mind is that often when people make silly or even rude comments about something, it's because they are unfamiliar and uncomfortable with it. It's easier for some to tease you than to just ask what it is you're eating. We've found that what works just as well as playing the cancer card (maybe even better) is to just smile and say, "No this is a really yummy quinoa salad. It gives me a lot of energy and tastes really good. Want to try some?" Sometimes they will and sometimes they won't.

When you're dealing with your immediate family, those who live and eat with you daily—be it your spouse, partner, significant other, children or parents—it's important to communicate openly about your goals in the kitchen and your diet. Explain why you're making the changes you are, that it's important to you and it would be wonderful if they could support you and give some of these foods a try themselves.

Children can be a tough audience with new foods, especially if you have picky eaters. Having a hard time getting your little ones (or maybe they aren't so little) to try some of your new culinary creations? You may need to be a little sneaky to make it work. Give some of these tips a try:

- Hide healthier foods in foods you know your kids will already eat. Make a fruit smoothie and add some leafy greens, like kale, to it. Purée up leafy greens or other veggies like carrots and zucchini and add to your spaghetti sauce. Add some fruit and nuts to your pancakes or shredded carrots and raisins to your muffins.

- Get your kids in the kitchen with you. How you do this varies depending on the age of your child, but kids often enjoy being helpful in the kitchen and feeling proud of something they created. Then, they will actually want to eat it! Younger kids love to make granola, smoothies and baked goods.

- Have a conversation with your older children, explaining why you are making some changes with food. Be open and honest and ask them if they will at least try some of these new foods. Show them how they can help and educate them on why these foods are better. You may find that your teenager wants to eat better too—seriously! We've taught healthier eating in high schools, and most of the students are very interested.

Embracing the Unfamiliar

TRYING NEW FOODS and new things in life means stepping outside of your comfort zone once in a while. Rather than fighting and struggling through change, learn to embrace it as a part of a life that will only make you a happier, more amazing person. Have fun with it and love yourself as you are getting healthier with these changes! Yeah, we know that some (or all) of what we're talking about might be new to you, but it's all super beneficial to your health and happiness. And know that these new foods are supporting your body and helping you fight cancer and other nasty stuff. Besides, seriously, if you've been given the cancer card, making some changes in your diet and life style is a piece of cake, comparatively speaking.

Here's one way to look at trading in your Big Mac for miso soup: It's one of the best things that will come out of your cancer status. A lot of the rest of it really sucks, but taking on a new food attitude and adapting your diet is only going to make you feel better physically, emotionally and mentally, because food is that power-ful. Here's what we've discovered: Food changes everything, and change can be delicious!

You also never know how the people around you may end up making their own changes with food. Most people want to be healthier, but it's figuring out how and getting inspired that becomes the tricky part. When we first began making changes in our diets, we did it for ourselves. And we learned that we're not just cooking, but we're also caring for our bodies and our lives. Later on, we also wanted to help others do the same and actually created a career out of that. The bonus? Our family and friends around us became pretty interested in our latest recipes and new foods. They started asking questions and incorporating some of the same new foods into their diets, and as they did they experienced more energy, better sleep, aches and pains disappeared and they lost weight. It became a ripple effect and we think that's pretty cool. So while you're taking on quinoa and kale, you just may be inspiring others as well.

Pantry Pals and Savvy Staples

————～～～～～————

IT'S PROBABLY CLEAR to you by now that we are all about getting in the kitchen and preparing clean, whole foods for optimal health. We try to do that whenever we can; however we also know that busy lives do not always make that possible or easy. That's why fast food is such a hit—it may not be good for you, but it's quick and easy, which fits in perfectly with our crazy schedules.

So, while we stress creating time for real food cooking and making that a priority in your life, we also need to be realistic. And of course, if you're dealing with cancer crap, you sometimes need food that comes in a package, but still supports your healthy eating goals. We have some favorite brands that can be found in our pantries, and want to share them with you. These are all packaged foods that are as close to the whole food as possible and are still nutrient-rich and health-boosting.

ALVARADO ST. BAKERY: This company offers sprouted and organic whole-wheat breads, bagels and tortillas that have delicious flavor. We like to keep their tortillas on hand in the fridge to use as a wrap for veggies, beans and rice, tempeh and more.

ANCIENT HARVEST QUINOA: Find whole grain quinoa in a box from this company, plus quinoa pastas and even polenta—all certified organic and gluten-free. If you're used to traditional white pasta, this pastas makes a nice substitute as it has a similar texture and flavor. You may want to add a tablespoon of olive oil to the water when cooking Ancient Harvest pasta to help prevent it from sticking together.

BOB'S RED MILL: This brand offers natural, gluten-free and certified organic products such as oats, flours, baking mixes like pancakes, whole grain cereals and even soup mixes.

BRAD'S RAW CHIPS: Called the "Healthiest Chips in the World," these tasty snacks come in a package, but offer pure, raw-food goodness. Try their kale, sun-dried tomato, hot red bell pepper and sweet-potato chips.

EXPLORE ASIAN AUTHENTIC CUISINE: Try these bean pastas (mung, soy and black bean) as an alternative to typical grain pastas.

EDEN ORGANIC: This organic brand includes canned goods without the use of BPA that can leach into food. Also try their tamari, sea veggies and teas.

FOOD FOR LIFE: This umbrella brand offers Ezekiel 4:9, Genesis 1:29 and Gluten-free breads, pasta, tortillas, English muffins and more. What's so wonderful about these? They are made with sprouted whole grains and no flour, which means they contain nutrient-rich living food, a big step up from "enriched" breads. The Ezekiel 4:9 products contain six sprouted grains and legumes that, when combined, make a complete protein.

LARA BAR: These are awesome whole-food bars made mostly with nuts and sweetened with dates. They come in a variety of flavors and are a perfect snack, full of protein.

LUNDBERG FAMILY FARMS: This family-owned company promotes sustainable farming practices. They offer gluten-free rice products: organic brown rice, rice cakes, rice chips, rice pastas, flour and brown-rice syrup.

MAINE COAST SEA VEGETABLES: Visit seaveg.com to order nutrient-rich, cancer-fighting sea veggies, if they are not sold locally in stores.

NAVITAS NATURALS: Find plenty of superfoods put into convenient packages by Navitas Naturals. Many powders and seeds are available that go nicely in smoothies, and we include several in our recipes. Try goji, acai, maca, cacao, chia seeds, hemp seeds, lucuma and wheatgrass.

TINKYADA RICE PASTA: You can find spaghetti, linguini, lasagna noodles, macaroni and other pasta types, all made from brown rice and gluten-free. Some are also certified organic.

TRADITIONAL MEDICINALS: These organic herbals teas not only warm you up, but also help to support, strengthen and heal your body.

———~~~~~———

We also have a suggested list of general, staple pantry and refrigerator items that make it easy to throw healthy, whole food meals together. You'll find most of these in our kitchens and in many of the recipes.

BEANS AND LENTILS: black beans, adzuki beans, green lentils, red lentils

CONDIMENTS: tamari, mirin (rice cooking wine), raw apple-cider vinegar, rice vinegar, honey

FRUIT AND VEGGIES: bananas, apples, berries, lemons, kale, lettuce mix, carrots, cabbage, sweet potato, onion, garlic

GRAINS: brown rice, quinoa, steel-cut or rolled oats, brown rice and quinoa pasta, sprouted grain wraps

NUT AND SEED BUTTERS: almond butter, peanut butter, tahini

NUTS, SEEDS AND DRIED FRUIT: almonds, walnuts, cashews, hemp seeds, sesame seeds, raisins, raw unsweetened coconut, dates

OILS: avocado, unrefined coconut, olive

OTHER: nutritional yeast, non-dairy milk, coconut water, herbal teas

PROTEINS FOR THE REFRIGERATOR: miso, tempeh, tofu

SEA VEGETABLES: kombu strips, shaker sea veggies

SPICES AND HERBS (DRY OR FRESH): cumin, curry powder, turmeric, oregano, ginger, thyme, rosemary

Putting It All Together

NOW YOU HAVE many of the tools needed to start eating well and feeling awesome as a result. We're going to take it a step further to help you pull everything together, using our recipes, guidelines and advice.

The first and probably the most important step you can take in improving your diet is adding in more veggies. How can you do that? There are so many ways to up your veggie intake! Try eating your veggies at breakfast. Sauté some zucchini, kale and garlic alongside your eggs or try our Curried-Tofu Breakfast Burrito (page 211). Plan your meal around your vegetable, so that it makes up most of your meal. Make a stir fry and add as many vegetables as you can to create a variety of textures and colors (and nutrients). Add veggies, like leafy greens, to your smoothies (try the Gorgeous Green Smoothie, page 198). Purée veggies, like beets, carrots and cauliflower, and mix into your baked goods (check out our Banana Veggie Muffins, page 216). Try a new vegetable every week—we've done this, and it's a lot of fun! Add veggies (try carrots, spinach, kale, zucchini, mushrooms and broccoli) to spaghetti sauce, your pizza and soups. Snack on carrot, celery and cucumber sticks with our Edamame Hummus (page 288). See? There are so many ways to get those veggies in—you just have to make the effort and make veggies a priority. It all happens in steps, and upping your plant foods takes time, commitment and a little planning.

Also remember that reducing the amount of animal food in your diet may take some getting used to as well as a different mind-set. Many of us are so used to having a big piece of chicken or slab of steak as the main part of our meal, often with a processed simple carbohydrate, like white pasta, and a small amount of vegetables on the side. Now it's time to reverse that thinking: Focus on your vegetables first, add in your whole grains and try eating more plant-based protein foods. If a typical dinner for you is one like we just described, start by adding in or increasing your vegetable portion. Then make some brown rice instead of the pasta. Next, try making tempeh instead of that chicken breast.

To get you going with your new food attitude and meal planning, we've supplied you with a three-day meal plan below. You can follow it exactly or make substitutions, but have fun with it and start nourishing that beautiful body! Particularly if you are going through some sort of cancer treatment right now, you may not be able to stomach certain meals or foods or you may feel the need for extra protein. Use this as a starting point and make changes as needed, so it works for you!

Day 1

BREAKFAST: Creamy Raspberry-Walnut Oatmeal (page 212), Vital Greens Tea (page 313)

SNACK: Banana Split Smoothie (page 202)

LUNCH: Curried Quinoa (page 252), veggie sticks with Edamame Hummus (page 288)

SNACK: Tasty Trail Mix (page 291)

DINNER: Creamy Broccoli Soup (page 278), Sweet and Strong Adzuki Beans (page 267)

Day 2

BREAKFAST: Gorgeous Green Smoothie (page 198),
Nutty Cranberry-Coconut Granola (page 214)

LUNCH: "Meaty" Bean Burgers (page 264)

SNACK: Quick Veggies and Delish Dips (page 294)

DINNER: Savory Stuffed Acorn Squash (page 232),
Cashew Kale (page 223)

DESSERT: Chocolate-Raspberry Mousse (page 298)

Day 3

BREAKFAST: Eggless Broccoli-Tomato Frittata (page 208)

SNACK: Crispy Kale Chips (page 285)

LUNCH: Tahini Spinach Spelt Berries (page 249),
Fennel String-Bean Salad (page 236)

SNACK: Mint Chocolate-Chip Smoothie (page 199)

DINNER: Mexican Bean Skillet (page 266), Arugula Salad with
Raspberry Vinaigrette (page 224), Brown Rice from
Whole Grain Cooking Chart (page 244)

CHAPTER 6

Chowing Down

Just when you were starting to feel all safe and snuggly in your new and improved food groove, you get invited out to dinner. Or have to travel. Or you are stuck hanging out in one of those cute (not!) hospital gowns for a while. What now? No need to panic! We've been there and will guide you through all these situations so you can make the healthiest food choices possible. We also have some helpful ideas to share around that other C-word: cravings! And who thought *how* you eat matters?! We'll share with you how to turn your mealtime into a healing, meditative practice.

On the Go

SURE, WE LOVE to be in the kitchen and cook yummy, healthy food for our bodies. But there are those times that, whether for work or pleasure, we want or need to eat out. And there are those days when we are on the go nonstop, running to appointments, or traveling near and far.

How do we make healthy food choices while out and about? The key is to do the best you can with the options you have. If you can choose between a drive-thru and a café, choose the café. If you have a gas station with candy versus a convenience store where you can create your own sandwich or salad, go for the store. Even when making the better choice requires a bit more effort, your body and mind will pay you back with more energy and better moods than if you just opt for convenience.

In gas stations, look for trail mix bars, nuts and seeds, or pretzels. In convenience stores there are more options—many have areas with prepared foods, often including veggies, salads, fruits and snacks. You may find a counter where you can create your own sub or entrée. For a beverage, reaching for water is best, or look for vegetable juice. Diet drinks with artificial sweeteners are, as we chatted about in Chapters 3 and 5, poor choices for saving calories or promoting health. If you find yourself in the drive-thru lane, opt for salads or a baked potato and steer clear of the fried, processed foods.

Planes are tricky, as it is often difficult to bring along food when traveling. Eat a nutrient-dense meal before takeoff and stash some healthy snacks in your bag. If you have time before your travels, check out some of our recipes, many of which are portable and can be tossed into a purse or taken along in a thermos or other container.

If you are eating out at a restaurant, here are some tips to keep in mind when placing your order:

- **DON'T DRINK YOUR CALORIES.** Cocktails, juice mixes and sodas fill us up with empty calories—which is another way of saying there's no nutrient bang for your caloric buck with these choices. It's not hard to down a drink or two while waiting for a meal and another while eating, so be mindful of the beverages you are choosing. Your best bet is sticking to water, seltzer or tea.

- **ACE THE APPETIZERS.** Whether you are munching mindlessly while chatting with your peeps or starving and can't wait for your entrée, appetizer time can be tricky. With the typical bread basket and the often highly processed hors d'oeuvres, the time between when you order and when your meal reaches your table can be precarious. For a healthier start, order a side salad, vegetable soup, or ask for raw veggies and some olive oil for drizzling.

- **CONTROL YOUR CONDIMENTS.** Restaurants are known for slathering on the dressings and oils, as well as seasonings like salt and sweeteners like sugar. Ask your server to put sauces or dressings on the side (be like Sally in the diner scene in *When Harry Met Sally*) so you can decide how much to use. Request your dish to be made with less or no salt, oil or sugar.

- **KEEP THINGS SIMPLE.** The simpler your food, the easier to know exactly what you are getting. Keeping things simple also means eating an appropriate portion size—not always easy to do in an era in which, especially in restaurants, portion sizes have greatly increased over the past generation. Consider sharing an entrée with a friend or ask to have half of your meal boxed to take home.

- **DOUBLE UP ON VEGGIES.** Ask for steamed, blanched or (if appropriate) raw veggies which can replace simple carbs (like white rice, white bread and pasta).

- **LOOK FOR LEAN PROTEIN.** If you are eating vegan, ask for beans, lentils or tofu. If you are incorporating some animal protein in your diet, look for eggs or fish. Ethnic restaurants often have a greater variety of choices in the protein and whole-grain categories (request, for example, brown rice instead of white).

Most importantly, don't be afraid to speak up and ask for what you want, even if it's not on the menu. Most places are happy to omit certain ingredients or make substitutions. If all else fails, you can pull out your Cancer Card and make your special request. And lastly, it goes without saying (but we'll say it anyway) that eating food regularly and frequently that you don't prepare yourself puts someone else in the driver's seat of your nutritional choices and of exactly what goes into your body. Of course we all need a break from the kitchen once in a while, so enjoy the opportunity to change things up and explore different foods.

Sick Food

WE'VE ALWAYS FOUND it astounding that—in a place dedicated to helping people get well and feel better—hospital food usually does just the opposite. You'll most likely have no problem ordering a hamburger and fries from your hospital menu card. But try to find some brown rice and kale! Unless you are lucky enough to receive care in one of the few forward-thinking hospitals that get the connection between

Living With the Questions

We can't hurry anything along by being angry, sad or impatient. Sometimes things take longer than we'd like or aren't as clear as we'd like. For those times, we've found it helpful to keep the following in mind (with apologies to Rainer Maria Rilke, for our adjustments): *"Have patience with everything unresolved in your heart and body and try to love the questions themselves as if they were locked rooms or books written in a very foreign language. Don't freak over the answers that are not given to you now, because you would not be able to live them. And the point is, to live everything. Live the questions now. Perhaps then, someday far in the future, you will gradually, without ever noticing it, live your way into the answer . . ."*

food and health, you'll need some creative solutions to solve the dilemma of what to eat when you are spending time there.

To have the most control over the food you are putting into your body in the hospital, the best idea is to arrange to bring your own food. Unless there are special circumstances, your medical team will most likely not have a problem with you providing your own chow. Of course if you are dealing with issues such as low white blood-cell count or taking certain medications that carry dietary restrictions, you will want to take those factors into account when planning your meals.

If you know you'll be spending time in the hospital, cook and store some nourishing foods ahead of time and have friends and family bring them when they visit. Or ask some peeps to cook for you using the recipes in this book, and then bring a hospital care-package to your room. Most likely, they will be happy to know there is something they can do to make your stay better. The nourishment and love you receive from supportive food will help you heal faster and get home quicker, so it is really worth the effort to arrange for healthy food during your stay.

Meals can be brought in thermoses to keep warm or cold, and in portable containers for storage. If items need to be kept cool or reheated, don't be afraid to ask the nurse if there is an area on the floor for patients to store and prepare food. If not, perhaps the staff room has a kitchenette you would be allowed to have access to, or where a nurse could reheat the food for you. Unfortunately this usually involves using a microwave, something we don't generally recommend. However, when faced with the necessity of spending time in the hospital, or anywhere that doesn't provide optimal food opportunities, we need to make the best choices possible in the situation and let go of the rest.

Kendall:

When I went into the hospital to have a sternotomy before I began chemotherapy, I hadn't begun to change my diet yet. I ate hospital food, including grilled-cheese sandwiches, white-flour pancakes, sugary Jello and ice cream. I think maybe I had a little broccoli, too.

When I went into the hospital three years later to give birth to my baby boy, I was fully prepared. I knew I needed the best, most nourishing food my body could get in that situation, and I wanted nothing less. I packed whole-food bars (the Lara Bar brand), kale chips, trail mix, granola and almond milk, bananas, apples, hummus and veggie sticks, tea bags and coconut water. We were able to store perishables in a small kitchen with a refrigerator. The hospital was also close by a healthier deli I knew of, and my husband purchased a couple of our meals there. It was so wonderful to have healthy food that made me feel good and helped give my body strength and support during a time when I really needed it!

Another approach for eating in the hospital is to find healthier options on the menu. While some hospitals sport fast-food franchises, others are getting with the groove and going healthy. Many facilities have signed the Healthy Food in Health Care pledge created by the international coalition Health Care Without Harm, and have committed to developing healthy food purchasing policies and systems. Some already have vegetarian, vegan and gluten-free options for their patients and staff, and include local and organic produce in their meals.

Even if you find yourself in a facility that doesn't prioritize healthy eating, it is usually possible to cobble together some options at mealtime. If you don't see what you are looking for on the printed menu, make sure to speak with a nurse or dietician to see if your request can be accommodated. Ask for salads, fresh fruit, and lightly steamed veggies. Choose whole grains if available and inquire if you can have a serving of beans or lentils. Perhaps there is a veggie burger or falafel-and-hummus pita available. Remember if you don't ask, you won't know, so speak up to see if your dietary needs can be met.

Healthy Options for Cravings

GOING THROUGH CANCER or not, we've all had encounters with cravings. Whether it is a piece of chocolate cake, a bag of potato chips or a cigarette, we tend to label anything we think we shouldn't consume, but often can't resist, as a craving. Cravings can be seen as a vice or weakness, a strong force against which we often seem powerless. However, consider for a moment the possibility that cravings might actually be an important way our bodies communicate with us and helps us achieve balance. When you experience a craving, instead of rushing in to satisfy it immediately, take a moment and try to understand it, to deconstruct it. Ask yourself, "What does my body want?" and "Why might it want that?" Even when we crave something we consider healthy, rather than naughty, there still may be a message behind it. Get curious and take a look at the foods, situations and behaviors in your life that are the underlying causes of your cravings.

Here are some possible reasons you might be experiencing cravings, to help get you started:

- Hormonal shifts like those during menstruation, pregnancy and menopause (also chemo-induced menopause) can cause unique food hankerings.

- The changing of the seasons or special holidays can make us yearn for specific foods.

- A longing for comfort, or even needing some TLC, may drive us to desire certain chow.

- Work that isn't personally meaningful and fulfilling may cause emotional eating and cravings to help fill a void.

- Stress, boredom or fatigue may be the reason we crave foods to soothe, entertain or energize.

- Indulging in one extreme in our foods, for example salty, can cause us to crave the opposite extreme, sweet, and vice versa.

If you notice any of these causes at the root of your craving, see if you can find another solution to the craving. Perhaps you can drink a glass of water and wait a bit to see if the craving subsides. Maybe you can work on eating foods more in the middle of the sweet-salty spectrum, such as grains, beans and veggies, and find some balance. You could call a friend, ask for a hug, or connect with others by writing or reading a blog, if what you are really craving isn't something that comes on a plate. Or perhaps you can try a healthier version of a traditional food you may be longing for at a certain time of the month or the year. Remembering that sweet potato-marshmallow-brown-sugar dish your aunt always made for Thanksgiving? Try a baked sweet potato with a drizzle of maple syrup.

Another cause for cravings can be missing nutrients. Often when our diets have been one-sided or lacking vitamins and minerals, we find ourselves faced with frequent food desires. There are actually nutritional reasons we may want certain chow. If you are craving sweets, for example, your body may be saying it is missing out on sulfur (try cranberries, cruciferous veggies, onions and garlic) or tryptophan (check out mustard greens, tofu, beans). When you are pining for oily snacks and fatty foods you may need more calcium (reach for kale, broccoli, dandelion greens or sesame seeds). Premenstrual cravings can be caused by a lack of zinc, so try green leafy veggies and root veggies.

Sometimes no matter what we do, we still have cravings for certain foods. Even then, we have a choice on just how "bad" we're really going to be. When you're clear on what you're craving, and you've ruled out other solutions—such as hydrating with a liquid or asking for a hug—see if you can "upgrade" your craving. If, for example, you're craving a banana split from your favorite ice-cream shop, try our Banana Split Smoothie (page 202). Desperate for chocolate? Try a small piece of high-quality dark chocolate, and savor. And make sure to check out the recipes in the cookbook section for some other terrific ideas.

Eating While Treating

CANCER TREATMENT CAN affect us in so many ways, all the way down to how our food tastes. It can create small and large changes in our appetite leading to weight gain or weight loss. Preparing for and recovering from surgery requires increased immune-system support and strategies for dealing with digestive sluggishness. Chemotherapy can cause mouth sores, making eating difficult if not nearly impossible. Chemo can also affect our sense of taste, leading to falling out of love with favorite foods and leaving us, quite literally, with a bad taste in our mouth. And radiation often results in tiredness and lack of energy.

In Chapter 7, "Eating for Support," you'll find specific foods and ideas to help with certain common concerns during and after cancer treatment. In this section we'd like to share with you some general advice around eating while treating.

If you've received a diagnosis and anticipate cancer treatment it's a smart idea to start planning ahead. Although you may not know exactly what you will be craving, or able to eat, you may want to do some food preparation. This can begin with stocking your pantry with some of your favorite go-to foods, as well as some of the ones we suggest in Chapter 7. You'll want to think of easy-to-grab foods when you may be hungry but don't feel like cooking. Be sure to check out the recipes in the cookbook under "Snack Time"—they're great for mini meals throughout the day or when you can only eat small portions at a time.

You will want to prepare some foods ahead of time that can be frozen for later use when you are not up to cooking. Soups, stews and broths are safe bets as are dishes like mashed sweet potatoes, veggie or bean burgers and healthy muffins. Make some granola (Nutty Cranberry-Coconut Granola; page 214), toss together a trail mix (Tasty Trail Mix; page 291) and freeze some oatmeal. You can also prep and chop fruits and veggies and store in the fridge. These can then be heated, used in smoothies, popped onto porridge, or stewed or baked. Having food ready and handy goes a long way to making sure you get the nutrition you need on those days during treatment when you are not able to spend much time in the kitchen.

For food storage we always recommend using glass if possible. You can freeze and reheat in glass Pyrex containers. Just make sure to allow some room for expansion before popping them in the freezer. If you do store food in plastic, make sure the food has cooled before placing it in the containers. Please do not heat or reheat food in plastic.

Chewing

Sure, we remember learning back in biology class that the digestive tract begins in the mouth. But have we ever stopped to think about what that really means? Or do we tend to see our mouth merely as the gulping gateway to our gut, or at most, the home of our taste buds, those little demons that drive us to want to devour all things sweet and salty? It might not be glamorous, but chewing our food thoroughly is actually one of the most beneficial things we can do for our body and our health. And, cross our hearts, it will pay us back by helping our bodies look glamorous!

Chewing our chow allows our brain to register when we are full and it satisfies our desire to chew. Slinging down food can be a reason we experience digestive issues such as reflux, IBS and (gasp!) gas. Chewing also gives our food more contact time with our enzyme-containing saliva, which helps to start breaking down the food as well, and improves digestion. Start by becoming aware of how many times you chew each mouthful of food, and then work on increasing the number of chews per bite. See if you can make it to 5, then 10, then 20, then 40, then 50. Of course we may not want to or be able to chew every bite of our meal 50 times. But when we make a commitment to chewing at least a portion of our meals well, we can begin to reap the benefits.

Another important step for eating while treating is getting support with cooking and meals. When you might need help and how much help you might need will depend on the individual circumstances of your treatment. At first it may be difficult to know, but once you begin any regular, recurring treatments, you will gain insight into how you will feel and how much support you would like. Maybe you just need a meal the day of treatment. Maybe meals for the days following treatment would be better. Or maybe you prefer to have some friends come and cook at your place.

A good piece of advice is to have one person organize and arrange meals for the times you have requested. She can take care of all the correspondence and arrangements, which allows you to save your energy and concentrate on healing, rather than logistics. Make sure to give the coordinator the names and numbers (or e-mail addresses) of friends and neighbors who might be willing to be part of the meal-delivery team, and also let her know your food preferences. Most people want to make food they know you will eat, so don't be shy about letting them know what you'd like. Most are also willing to try a new dish, so feel free to ask your coordinator to give them your favorite recipe (or this book!) when it is their turn to cook.

And as a side note: Do not feel obligated to eat everything a friend or family member brings for you if it is not your cup of tea or you don't feel it would be best for your health. Oftentimes well-meaning people associate caring for others with providing sweets, cookies, cupcakes, anything to help a friend or family member "feel better," a culinary Band-Aid for the boo-boo. While it can be fine to have a treat every once in awhile if your condition allows, a continual procession of goodies streaming into your home from well-meaning peeps is not supportive of your health. Even if you have to give certain items the toss, it is more important that you eat what you want and need rather than chowing down on food you don't enjoy or is just plain bad for you.

Eating while treating will require listening to your body and making adjustments as you go. But don't be hard on yourself if you have days in which you are happy to have gotten anything down, nutritious or not! Experiment with different, supportive foods, as well as size and frequency of meals and snacks. And one final girlfriend tried-and-true tip: Visualize the food you are taking into your body powerfully supporting you and all the cells in your body with all of its cancer-kicking goodness.

Get Your Zen On

~~~~~~~~~~~~~~

SO OFTEN AROUND cancer, we find ourselves entrenched in worry, anxiety, sadness and pain. We've been there (heck, we still end up there sometimes!) and know just how overwhelming that can be.

There is much that can be scary, since there are often a lot of unknowns, and it isn't hard to allow your mind to carry you away with thoughts and ideas about what is happening or what might happen. All the while you may be sitting in a chair, lying

Let's Talk About Sex

In case you didn't notice, cancer can really throw your love life for a loop. But you're unlikely to hear your oncologist or surgeon say the words, "Let's talk about sex." So you might think you'll just have to deal with one more way this nasty disease has changed your life for the worse. Cancer can leave you stressed and fatigued. Add the effects of chemo and radiation and the aftermath of surgery and, possibly, a transformed body, and it's no wonder you're likely to be feeling anything but "in the mood."

The good news is you don't have to give up your love life just because you're dealing with cancer. Find the support you need by looking for a sexual health and medicine specialist, preferably someone who has experience working with women dealing with cancer. There are also organizations such as the Center for Intimacy After Cancer Therapy and others that offer books and therapists to guide you in reclaiming your lost sexual mojo and expanding your intimacy repertoire.

in a bed, or talking to a friend. But are you there? Or are you actually not sitting in that chair, not lying in that bed, not mindfully talking to that friend, but rather hanging out in the universe called Worst Case Scenario and missing out on the moment and, therefore, on your life?

How to get back to the present? One approach is by training in the practice of mindfulness. What is mindfulness? It means paying attention—but not in an intellectual, thinking kind of way. Rather, mindfulness implies a noticing of *what is* that is not judging, comparing or analyzing. It is the opposite of our typical state of preoccupation in which our mind avoids abiding in the now and follows thoughts as a hunting dog darts after the trail of a rabbit. This common mode of living and being separates you from your immediate experience and, far from protecting you and making you happy, leads to sadness, feelings of isolation and depression. And, what's particularly tragic: Until you become aware of this habit, you don't even notice. When you realize you don't have to be at the mercy of your thoughts, when you experience that you needn't allow your mind to carry you away with memories, stories and hypothetical "what ifs," when you simply place your attention lightly, intentionally and bravely on the present moment and accept it just as it is, you can experience inner resources of strength, wisdom and peace.

How can you do this? One way to cultivate mindfulness is through the practice of meditation (read more about meditation in Chapter 8). Another—and our favorite—is through cooking and eating mindfully.

Are you present and cooking when you are cooking? Do you even realize you are chewing when you are chewing? Spending time with food, both in preparing it and eating it, gives us the chance to really come into the moment and connect with the experience using all of our senses. It is an opportunity to slow down, take a "time out" and just focus on nourishing body, mind and spirit.

When we accept the idea that the food we choose to eat, the spirit in which it

Annette:

I made the decision (and it was one I had to commit to time and time again) that, since I had this crappy cancer diagnosis and my life might be cut short, I was not going to waste what time I did have continually analyzing all the potential "what ifs." I could either be present for my life—in whatever shape and for however long that might be—or I could be stuck in worry, fear and dread. That last option sounded to me like the "might as well already be dead" option, so I decided to be in the now, as best I could, in whatever moments I had. This decision doesn't require anything remotely related to sainthood, it just takes a commitment to show up for life, moment by moment, however it appears. In my experience there is power, strength, joy (believe it or not!) and also peace to be found in making this commitment and fostering this awareness in your life.

is prepared and the atmosphere and manner in which we take the food into our bodies matters, then mealtime ceases to be merely an exercise in the easiest and fastest way to fill a hole in our stomach. We are caring for our body, for our life, when we are present while we cook and while we eat.

We didn't believe until we tried it, but there is nothing like working with real food to bring a sense of calm and centeredness into your being. If you give yourself fully to the task, enjoying the colors, textures, aromas, tastes and sounds of the kitchen becomes an opportunity to connect with all of your senses, and with life-supporting nature and abundance. There are moments and days when this will be more challenging than others. The key is persistence—doing the best you can at each moment and dropping any judgment of what might constitute "slipping up"—as you continually commit anew to being present while you care for yourself in the kitchen.

As an extra bonus, eating food prepared with attention nourishes your body and spirit. Think about how your body feels after eating industrially produced fast food consumed in the car or in front of the computer. Now think about how it feels after eating a thoughtfully prepared home-cooked meal shared with family or friends. Taking the time to cook, eating in a peaceful atmosphere and chewing food thoroughly all contribute to your well-being, anchor you in the moment and help you not only to be present for but also to enjoy your life.

Practicing Patience

————◦◦◦◦◦◦◦◦◦◦◦◦————

WHEN WE ARE stuck in Cancer World the concept of patience is, well, challenging. We just want to get the heck out of here, ASAP. We want information gathered, decisions made, progress shown, our future clear . . . *now.*

Especially if we are used to plotting our lives in every detail, checking off our to-do lists and having things pretty much *under control*, being caught off guard by cancer can throw the proverbial monkey wrench into our best-laid plans. Cancer shows us quite clearly that we will probably be forced to live with much that is unknown, both short-term and long-term. We will want answers when there aren't any (yet). We will want to know that we will continue to be here (which our doctors can't promise us, with or without cancer). We will want our hair to grow quicker, our scars to heal faster, our bodies to get healthier more rapidly.

In the meantime, if you're like us, you'll want to slug whoever that smartass was who came up with the saying that patience is a virtue. Hard as it is to accept, the smartass had a point, and a pretty good one. Sometimes, after we have done all we can, the best thing we can do is to try our best to relax and be patient. The problem is, we are so convinced we have to "do something." But when we cultivate patience and create spaciousness, something comes in to fill this space. This "something" is often wisdom, intuition, answers, insight.

CHAPTER 7

Eating for Support

N ow that you know what types of foods are crucial for a healthy body and soul—whether you have cancer or not—we want to make sure you have the food arsenal to really kick ass with cancer, during treatment and beyond. And we want you to understand why these foods are important. These are the foods that can help support and protect certain organs and systems in your body, and will be useful should cancer rear its ugly face again.

We've also made it really easy for you: Each recipe in the cookbook section lists its specific benefits, letting you know which are helpful in soothing side effects or supporting different body systems and functions. Need to fight fatigue? Want to help boost blood-cell production? There's a recipe for that! Plus we've listed some sample recipes with page numbers after each section in this chapter. See? Easy!

Blood

EATING FOODS THAT support the blood is very important because blood is pumping through every inch of your body, bringing nutrients and oxygen to organs, bones, muscles, skin, tissues and cells. And how do those nutrients get into your blood? Here's a quick reminder of how the digestive system works, in a nutshell. You take a bite of food and chew it up. That food travels down your esophagus to your stomach where it is broken down by digestive juices. It then travels into the intestines where more digestive juices break the food down further before it is absorbed through the intestinal walls into—you guessed it—the bloodstream.

When dealing with cancer, our blood cells can become overproduced or underproduced, due to the cancer itself or side effects of treatment. Particularly during chemotherapy, it can be challenging to keep the red and white blood-cell counts within a healthy range. A low red blood-cell count can lead to anemia, which causes weakness and fatigue. A low white blood-cell count can lead to neutropenia. Neutropenia is a condition in which the number of neutrophils—one type of white blood cell—is decreased. When this happens, the immune system is weak and has a tougher time fighting off infection. Your doctor will most likely prescribe a medication to boost blood cell production (and you'll know it's working when your bones ache, because those blood cells are being produced in overdrive by your bone marrow). However, you can help alter the production of blood cells in the bone marrow and help build strong, healthy blood by eating blood-boosting foods. You can also eat food that helps to cleanse toxins from the blood.

One major blood-boosting food group is sea vegetables such as wakame, nori, alaria and kombu (kelp). Sea veggies, or seaweed, help rebuild and support blood cells. We offer a couple of delicious sea vegetable recipes in this book, but you can also purchase sea veggies in shakers and add to soups, salads, rice and veggies as you would salt or pepper. As we mentioned earlier, one easy way to get your superfood sea veggies is by adding a six-inch strip of kombu to your pot of rice or beans as they cook. The nutrients from the kombu will be absorbed into your food.

Foods rich in beta-carotene and other carotenes strengthen white blood-cell production, resulting in a stronger immune system. These include yellow, orange and red veggies like carrots, bell peppers and beets, as well as dark leafy greens such as kale, spinach and collards. Other white blood cell boosters include spirulina (blue-green algae available in capsule and powder form), burdock, garlic, almonds and navy beans.

In the Recipes

Blood-boosting recipes include Dandelion Greens With Warm Tahini Dressing (page 220), Cool Collard Green Slaw (page 222), Cashew Kale (page 223), Good Luck

Greens (page 225), Nori Veggie Rolls (page 231), Arame Red Cabbage Salad (page 237), Burdock and Carrot Sauté (page 238), Hearty Navy-Bean Vegetable Stew (page 260), Carrot-Beet Juice (page 310) and Krazy Kale Juice (page 311).

Brain

——~~~~~~~~——

IT CAN BE tough to maintain mental clarity on a daily basis with the busy lives so many of us lead: From heavy workloads within our jobs to hectic days (and some sleepless nights) with kids, we often can't seem to think straight from being over-tired or stressed out. Add a poor diet to this equation and your brainpower could go downhill fast. Forgetfulness, confusion, memory loss, mood swings and inability to focus are not uncommon for people of all ages. Have you ever walked into a room and forgot why you were going there in the first place? Have you ever driven away with your cup of coffee sitting on the roof of your car? You're not the only one.

On top of that, if you've been treated with chemotherapy, you may suffer from "chemo brain." This term is used to describe memory loss and decreased mental clarity after cancer treatment, and many cancer peeps—including us! - declare they suffer or have suffered from it. While some say chemo brain doesn't really exist or that it is simply a result of emotional trauma, some research shows the contrary, although it's not completely clear if this side effect is actually from chemotherapy, other cancer treatment or cancer itself. A study conducted at the Stanford University School of Medicine in California showed that women who underwent chemotherapy had significantly less activity in the parts of the brain that are used for executive function (planning), cognitive control and monitoring as compared to women who had surgery and other treatments or women without cancer.[3]

Fortunately, simple improvements in diet and lifestyle can make significant and often immediate changes. Chowing down on brain-healthy foods like leafy greens and walnuts just might clear up that foggy head. Other brain-boosting foods include mono- and polyunsaturated fats like olive, flax seed, sesame, walnut, coconut, peanut oils (and fish, if you choose to consume it). Antioxidant-rich foods (berries, beans, artichoke hearts, pecans and hazelnuts) and B-vitamin foods (chickpeas, bananas, sweet potato, pinto beans, tahini, mushrooms, brown rice and eggs) are all important for brain health. And of course, getting enough sleep, water and challenging yourself with physical and mental exercise will also support your brain.

In the Recipes

Brain-boosting recipes include Super Berry Booster Smoothie (page 203), Creamy Raspberry-Walnut Oatmeal (page 212), Dandelion Greens with Warm Tahini Dressing (page 220), Sweet Potato Fries with Peanut Dipping Sauce (page 240), Cranberry Brown-Rice Pilaf (page 253), "Meaty" Bean Burgers (page 264), Walnut Meat-less Balls (page 269), Mighty Mushroom Soup (page 275), Sweet and Creamy Tomato Soup (page 280), Tasty Trail Mix (page 291) and Green Tea-Mango Sorbet (page 306).

Detoxifying

THE BODY NEEDS to release large amounts of waste products daily from its systems. The lungs, skin, kidneys and bowels are the four main channels of elimination. Each of these organs should ideally release two pounds of toxins per day. The liver is also an important part of your body's detox system; however, when the other four organs are detoxifying properly, the liver can spend more time on its other job: regulating metabolism. All of these systems must be in proper working order, and when one of them is functioning at lower levels, it puts an extra burden on the others. As a result, toxins can build up and lead to low energy and illness.

To help your body detoxify, you can try to reduce toxins going in and to help toxins going out. Toxins going in come from foods we eat that are highly processed, sprayed with pesticides or include other chemicals and dyes. Besides food, toxins also come from stress and environmental pollutants like cigarette smoke, automobile exhaust and swimming-pool chemicals.

You can also eat cleansing and fiber-rich foods and drink plenty of water to help those toxins leave the body. Water is crucial to life in general and allows the body to remove toxins through the skin and the kidneys. You can't flush those toxins out without plenty of water, so drink up. You've read about many of these wonderfully cleansing foods in other chapters, and they include leafy greens, daikon radish, onion, garlic, burdock root, millet, barley, kidney beans, water chestnuts, cranberries and blueberries. Fruits and vegetables, in general, contain fiber and water, so add plenty of those to your diet. Milk thistle is also detoxifying and supports liver function, and it can often be found as a tincture (just add drops to water) or a tea. Sea vegetables, chlorella and spirulina all have tremendous detoxifying benefits. Sea veggies can be added to salads, soups or rolled into sushi, and you'll find a few recipes using sea veggies in The Recipes section. Chlorella and spirulina can be taken in capsule or powder form. Try adding the powders to smoothies. Chlorella actually binds to heavy metals in the body and pulls them out in elimination.

As we mentioned earlier in Chapter 4, juicing occasionally can help to pull toxins from cells and get them moving out of the body. Just remember that on a regular basis your body still needs the fiber that is removed in juicing to keep waste elimination regular. Therefore juicing without eating any fiber-rich foods in your diet for any extended period of time is not advisable and may cause constipation. Try juicing occasionally or even once a day, while still incorporating whole, plant-based foods.

In the Recipes

Detoxifying recipes include Gorgeous Green Smoothie (page 198), Gingered Mustard Greens (page 221), Arugula Salad with Raspberry Vinaigrette (page 224), Good Luck Greens (page 225), Nori Veggie Rolls (page 231), Arame Red-Cabbage Salad (page 237), Burdock and Carrot Sauté (page 238), Millet Black-Bean Fritters (page 254), "Meaty" Bean Burgers (page 264), Blueberry Lemonade (page 309), Carrot-Beet Juice (page 310), Krazy Kale Juice (page 311) and Vital Greens Tea (page 313).

Respiratory

~~~~~~~~~~

EVEN IF THE cancer you are facing has nothing to do with your respiratory system, your treatment, particularly chemotherapy, may directly affect it, possibly causing damage to the lungs. Usually, for this reason, your oncologist will request a lung-function test before chemo begins to make sure your lungs are strong enough to take on chemo. You may even notice during chemo that your breathing is somewhat uncomfortable (or you may not notice at all). Knowing how you can help to strengthen your respiratory system can go a long way in helping to keep your breath strong and those lungs clear. Remember that your respiratory system is responsible for carrying oxygen to your blood, and healthy, well-oxygenated blood means a healthier, stronger body.

Foods that support the respiratory system include warm liquids like teas, broths and even warm water. These can help soothe the throat and flush toxins and mucous out of the body faster. Including antioxidant-rich foods, especially those with vitamin C, can help alleviate inflammation in the respiratory system. Stock up on leafy greens, fennel, papaya, red bell pepper, citrus fruit and cabbages. Another supporter is sea veggies because they are so nutrient-rich and detoxifying. Fortunately, all of these foods help your body in many ways, so you can add them in and do your entire body some serious good.

In the Recipes

Respiratory-supportive recipes include Cabbage and Cannellini Bean Sauté (page 219), Gingered Mustard Greens (page 221), Garlic Lover's Kale (page 226), Fennel String-Bean Salad (page 236), Arame Red-Cabbage Salad (page 237), Vegetable Stock (page 271), Mineral Stock (page 272), Blueberry Lemonade (page 309), Vital Greens Tea (page 313) and Sweet Ginger Tea (page 314).

Hormones and Endocrine System

CANCER TREATMENT CAN affect your endocrine system and hormones in several different ways. Chemotherapy can stop the ovaries from producing estrogen and progesterone. This may make your periods irregular or even cause temporary menopause until treatment is finished. (And you may wish to discuss fertility concerns with your oncologist before you begin treatment.) Radiation in the pelvic region may have the same effect. Radiation on or surgical removal of any part of the

Embrace Your Creativity

There's nothing like letting your creative side loose as a form of therapy. Only it doesn't need to feel like therapy. Cancer and life in general can build up some crazy emotions, and it's up to us to find a way to release and express them. Having some creativity in your life can serve you well. You don't have to be Claude Monet to do some painting. It doesn't need to be spectacular; just have fun with it and see what comes out on paper. Other terrific ways to get your creative juices flowing? Try writing, gardening, scrapbooking, knitting, cooking, redecorating a room in your home or playing a musical instrument.

endocrine system may result in hormonal imbalance. For example, if the ovaries are surgically removed, this will cause a sudden drop in estrogen levels. Breast and ovarian cancer treatment drugs, such as tamoxifen, a selective estrogen receptor modulator, can affect hormones and may create menopause symptoms like hot flashes.

So you see, as if having cancer and feeling sick from treatment wasn't enough, you also may have to deal with these lovely hormonal side effects. But the good news is that what you eat can help.

One superfood that helps to nourish the endocrine system and balance hormones is maca root. Maca has been used effectively for menopause, perimenopause, hot flashes, PMS and even fertility enhancement. Maca regulates hormones as it acts on the hypothalymus-pituitary gland. It can be purchased in supplement capsule form or as a powder that can be added to smoothies and cereals. Whole soy foods can also be helpful in balancing hormones and assist with hot flashes and PMS. Try eating soy foods like edamame (the soy bean), miso, tempeh and tofu.

You will most likely find that there isn't a "magic" food (although maca is pretty good stuff) that will fix those hormones. If you eat as we've been suggesting, with plenty of leafy greens, sea veggies, plant protein and whole grains and stay away from highly processed foods, refined sugars and too much animal protein (especially dairy) you will feel more balanced. Even outside of Cancer World, when you're eating this way, you'll probably notice fewer PMS or menopausal symptoms.

In the Recipes

Hormone-balancing recipes include Chocolate Malt Smoothie (page 196), Gorgeous Green Smoothie (page 198), Eggless Broccoli-Tomato Frittata (page 208), Garlic Lover's Kale (page 226), Marinated Tempeh Cutlets (page 259), Tempeh Salad (page 263), Edamame Hummus (page 288), Coconut Goji Energy Bars (page 292) and Creamy Veggie Goodness Dip (page 295).

Adrenals and Fatigue

THE ADRENAL GLANDS are part of the endocrine system and are located on the top of both kidneys. They are responsible for producing essential hormones, such as aldosterone, which regulates blood pressure, and cortisol, which regulates metabolism and helps the body respond to stress. Adrenaline is also created through the adrenals, and that hormone helps the body react to that stress. And since stress and cancer pretty much go hand in hand, your adrenals can really take a hit.

Even if you aren't fighting cancer, just the craziness of daily life can make you tired and stressed. Then we drink plenty of coffee and eat empty carbs that don't support our bodies but give us a quick pick-me-up followed by a crash later. It can be an endless cycle, and an important one to break.

If you are constantly experiencing stress and taking on more than these small glands can handle, you may feel run down, irritable and just plain exhausted. Long-term adrenal imbalance can lead to chronic fatigue and your adrenals and entire body will suffer. Fortunately the food you eat can be a big help in healing the adrenal glands. That and some deep breathing, yoga and a bubble bath—seriously!

Gluten, caffeine and sugar can be rough on the adrenals, so it would be wise to reduce or eliminate these types of foods. If you just can't skip your morning cup of coffee, be sure to eat a meal full of complex carbohydrates, like steel-cut oats or granola with nuts and berries. And as always, avoid processed foods, which can really wreak havoc on your adrenals. Keeping to food that we have discussed throughout this book—real, whole foods, and mostly plants—is what your body needs for optimal energy levels. We don't want you to add to your stress about how to prepare these amazing whole foods, so we provided all sorts of fabulous recipes in this book.

If you are looking for more adrenal support, try herbs like ashwagandha, licorice root and Siberian ginseng. These can often be found in tincture form and can be added to tea or warm water.

One other important piece to maintaining balanced adrenals is not just what you eat, but *when* and *how*. Be sure to balance your meals throughout the day and eat regularly. Eat breakfast within an hour of waking in the morning, to help restore your body's blood sugar levels. Don't skip lunch, and include midmorning and midafternoon snack if you're hungry. Include a light dinner—don't stuff yourself, but make sure you feel satisfied—and try not to eat later than 7pm. And what about *how* to eat? Sit down, take your time, chew your food slowly and really taste it, like we talked about in Chapter 6. Eat in a peaceful setting without the TV blaring, and try to stay off your computer. The more relaxed the environment you create when eating, the happier your adrenals—and you—will be.

On top of that, do not underestimate the importance of a good night's sleep and a catnap here and there—*especially* if you're fighting cancer! Your body does its best healing while at rest; when you're overtired, your immune system can't function optimally. Exercise is another key part of staying energized and of healthy adrenal function. Do whatever you can to get some movement into your day. It doesn't need to be a five-mile run. Walk up the block and back. Take a ride on your bicycle. Take the stairs instead of the elevator. If you can do more and do it regularly, please do! Your body will feel the difference, even if it's tough to get yourself going at first. And it *will* actually give you more energy.

In the Recipes

Fatigue-fighting recipes include Oatmeal-Carrot Cookie Smoothie (page 195), Superfood Smoothie (page 200), Simple Cinnamon Kasha (page 207), Creamy Raspberry-Walnut Oatmeal (page 212), Cashew Kale (page 223), Quinoa with Pears and Maple Vinaigrette (page 245), Tahini Spinach Spelt Berries (page 249), Cranberry

Brown-Rice Pilaf (page 253), Navy Bean Stew (page 260), Sweet and Strong Adzuki Beans (page 267), Tamari-Infused Tofu on Braised Bok Choy (page 268), Tasty Trail Mix (page 291) and Coconut Goji Energy Bars (page 292).

Immune System

HAVING A STRONG immune system is vital in fighting off bacteria, parasites and viruses, from cancer to the common cold, as well as aiding the body in excreting toxins. When the body gets run down from stress, lack of sleep and poor eating habits it affects the immune system, and as a result all of these organisms can more easily enter and take up residence in your body.

When you have cancer, it's important to support your immune system to help your body fight the disease. Cancer is a result of a "bad" cell multiplying at a rapid rate. Most people have some amount of cancerous cells in their bodies, but with a strong immune system, they are able to keep them from multiplying and growing enough to become a problem, which is when a tumor is detected.

What causes these cells to reproduce uncontrollably? And why do we have any cancer cells at all? Every day we are exposed to toxins in the air, in our food and even from stress. (We explained this earlier in this chapter, then talked about why it's important to detoxify the body.) As a result of this toxic exposure, cells can become damaged. The amount of damage and the number of cells affected depends on several factors including genetic makeup, the body's ability to remove those toxins on a daily basis and how many toxins enter the body in the first place. That's why it's important to limit the toxins going in (eat organic, clean, whole plant-based foods, get sleep, find ways to de-stress, be active) and help the toxins going out (we give you lots of good ideas for this under the "Detoxifying" section in this chapter).

So you can see that your body can't put up a proper fight without the right tools, which includes a kick-ass immune system. Supporting the immune system means exactly what we have been hammering into your beautiful head throughout this book: significantly reducing or eliminating refined sugars, animal foods and highly processed foods, and eating a plant-based, whole foods diet. Pay special attention to sea vegetables, leafy greens and water—get these immune boosters in whenever you can!

Other edible options we love are astragalus root, mushrooms and vitamin D. Astragalus can be found in capsule form, tincture or as a tea. It can also be purchased dried and added to mineral broths and soups. Mushrooms, such as reiki, shiitake and cordyceps can be eaten whole (the best way), sipped as tea or taken in capsule form. Vitamin D is best from the sun or can be taken as a supplement, which is available in capsule or liquid drop forms.

In the Recipes

Immune-boosting recipes include Superfood Smoothie (page 200), Super Berry Booster Smoothie (page 203), Dandelion Greens with Tahini Dressing (page 220), Garlic Lover's Kale (page 226), Baby Bok Choy with Shiitakes, Pumpkin Seeds and Gojis (page 227), Steamed Sesame Broccoli (page 235), Arame Red-Cabbage Salad (page 237) and Mighty Mushroom Soup (page 275).

Constipation

ANOTHER UNFORTUNATE SIDE effect of cancer treatment (mostly chemotherapy and surgery) is constipation. Yup, the ol' pooper can get quite plugged up. Your doctor will likely recommend taking a stool softener. Whether or not you opt to do that is up to you, but either way it would be helpful to be eating foods high in fiber and drinking plenty of water.

Let's make this easy so you don't stress about counting how many grams of fiber are in every food you eat. If you are eating the whole grains, vegetables, fruit and proteins we talk about, you should be getting plenty of fiber. However, if you do need to up your intake, try eating more of the following foods. For fruit it's easy: Just think of the letter P for prunes, papaya, pineapple, pears and peaches. Also figs and apricots. Get your fruit dried, fresh or add to smoothies. Other fiber-rich foods include broccoli, cabbage, brussels sprouts, chard, spinach, kale and squash. Sometimes it's easier on our digestive systems to eat these veggies cooked rather than raw. Beans and whole grains are also quite fiber-rich, particularly garbanzo, pinto and kidney beans and millet, brown rice and barley. Another fiber-friendly food: flax seed. Use ground flax seed in smoothies, on cereals and as a salad topping.

Keep in mind that if you aren't getting enough water, these high-fiber foods aren't going to work as well. Fiber works with water to make your stools soft, so drink up, eat up and get things moving!

In the Recipes

Constipation-kicking recipes include Cabbage and Cannellini Bean Sauté (page 219), Cashew Kale (page 223), Savory Stuffed Acorn Squash (page 232), Fennel String-Bean Salad (page 236), Fiesta Brown-Rice (page 246), Curried Quinoa (page 252), Creamy Broccoli Soup (page 278) and Almond Mylk (page 318).

Headaches

HEADACHES CAN BE prevalent during cancer treatment for various reasons. The chemo cocktail you may be receiving is full of powerful drugs that can cause dehydration and imbalance in your body, leading to headaches. You also may not be sleeping well or feel stressed. (Really? Stress and cancer? No way!) Or perhaps you had a recent cry-fest (yes, let it out!) and your head is pounding from that.

When your head is throbbing, remember you have that pain for a reason, and it's your job to figure out what that reason is. Below are some possible causes and corresponding treatment options for you to try.

- Drink water. Dehydration is common for many of us, even without that added bonus of chemotherapy or other medications related to cancer treatment. Be sure to drink your water constantly to help avoid the headaches that often come with dehydration.

- Drink electrolytes. If you've had diarrhea, have been vomiting or having night sweats (all common side effects of cancer treatment and sometimes of cancer itself), you lose not only water from your body, but also important vitamins and minerals needed to keep your body in balance. This loss of electrolytes can create some splitting headaches! Be sure to grab a healthy, natural electrolyte source. Stay far away from those sport and power drinks, like Gatorade or Powerade, that make claims of being good for you: Many of them have added dyes and are made up of artificial ingredients. Our favorite liquid source of electrolytes is all-natural coconut water. This stuff is fabulous and there is nothing added—it's simply the juice from the coconut. It contains dozens of electrolytes naturally, which will help to restore your body, so stock up and drink up!

• Lack of nutrients can cause your head to ache, so it's important to get in many of the nutrient-rich whole foods we discuss in this book. If your diet consists of pizza, bagels and ice cream, your body is not getting what it needs to fight cancer and feel as good as possible during the cancer craziness. Even if you aren't facing cancer, your body still needs those whole grains, veggies and plant-based proteins to stay strong, function properly and be able to fight off any disease that comes your way.

• Be sure you're getting enough food. If you aren't consuming enough calories, you will feel run down, your immune system will weaken and yes, you can also get a nasty headache. Unfortunately, eating can sometimes be tough with cancer treatment, if you're suffering from soreness in the mouth or throat area from radiation therapy, or nausea or mouth sores from chemotherapy, or just general lack of appetite. Look for the notes directly under each recipe title to find foods that are easier to eat when dealing with your specific treatment side effects.

• Release stress through massage, a walk, meditation, deep breathing, quiet time, a hot bath or any other way you think will help you relieve some tension. When we get stressed out, headaches often follow and sometimes the only way to relieve them is to take some time for you and be mellow.

Kendall:

I lived on coconut water during chemotherapy, and it helped me so much. Not only did it help to hydrate me, but it also restored the electrolyte balance in my body. Now, whenever I feel off balance after a workout, when I've sweat a lot or have a headache, I down a glass of it. I highly recommend it!

In the Recipes

Deyhdration-defending recipes include Blueberry Lemonade (page 309), Watermelon Slushie (page 312), Cool Cucumber-Mint Water (page 315) and Citrus Spritzer (page 317).

Nausea

———~~~~~~———

OH NAUSEA, HOW we despise thee. Let us count the ways. This is a common and very unpleasant side effect from chemo. Just when we need to feed our bodies plenty of nutrient-rich calories because we're in for the fight of our lives, suddenly we can't eat a darn thing. Foods you once loved now make you gag, sometimes just from the smell. Sometimes even the tasteless taste of water can leave you feeling ready to lose your lunch!

Nausea was one of the worst side effects for us, and there were certainly days when we just couldn't get much food down. However, it's important to find foods you can stomach to help keep your strength up, support your immune system and heal your body. This can be different for everyone and may even change for you from one week to the next.

One of the best tips we can give you is to not stress too much about the food you can manage to get down. If it happens to be a not-so-healthy choice at times, it's okay. Sometimes you gotta do what you gotta do. Just remember to try to get the good stuff in when you can and look for healthier alternatives to the foods that seem to work for you. For example, if ice cream seems to go down easily and soothes your sore mouth or throat, try eating our version of Coconut Ice Kreme (page 303), which omits the dairy and sugar, two foods you don't want to be eating when you're in the cancer seat.

In the Recipes

Nausea-nixing recipes include suggestions such as Berry Almond Smoothie (page 201), Gingerly Carrot Soup (page 274), Potato Leek Soup (page 277), Coconut Ice Kreme with Cherry Swirl (page 303), Watermelon Slushie (page 312), Sweet Ginger Tea (page 314) and Cool Cucumber-Mint Water with Raspberry Ice (page 315).

Weight Loss or Gain

CANCER TREATMENT IS a funny thing when it comes to your weight. If you have a tough time keeping food down due to nausea or just the stress of fighting cancer, you could start losing weight. And while this may seem like a surprise gift from the cancer gods, it's really not the way to drop those pounds. Sure, a few here and there isn't anything to worry about, but just remember you need as much nutrient-dense food as you can get to fight that cancer and keep your strength up, so it's helpful to eat foods high in protein and good fats. And no, these fats are not going to *make* you fat. Your body needs those healthy fats right now (actually you need them all the time), so don't be shy. Fill up on favorite fat foods including avocado (perfect in a smoothie), olive oil, olives, coconut oil, coconut, nuts and nut butters and sweet potatoes.

Protein pleasers like beans, nuts, nut butters, lentils, miso, tempeh, tofu, eggs in moderation and quinoa are all good choices. It's important to get more protein into your diet during cancer treatment not only to avoid losing too much weight and wasting away, but also to help your body repair and heal. Protein is needed to accomplish this: As you can imagine, your body is working overtime on some serious repairs!

Another reason to eat these calorie-dense foods is because they help to keep your energy up. You get more bang for your caloric buck with these foods, meaning you can eat less of them but still get plenty of nutrients and calories to sustain you.

Treatment can also lead to weight gain. Sometimes treatment includes the use of steroids, antidepressants or other drugs that can cause pounds to add up. Also, most people who are in cancer treatment are less active because they are weaker or just feel plain sick and don't want to get off the couch. Or you may be recovering from surgery and have limited mobility. This decrease in movement can result in weight gain. On top of that, dealing with cancer crap might bring out the emotional eater in you, and you may find there are days when all you want to do is drown your sorrows in a bag of cookies. Or maybe you've decided, "Hey, I have friggin' cancer. I'm going to eat whatever the heck I want." Oh, and then there's stress, of course. That can lead to extra pounds, too.

If weight gain has become a concern for you, you're already taking your first step by reading this book. Just make small changes in your diet, step by step, using our suggestions. And if you do that, you really shouldn't need to count calories religiously and instead can enjoy some amazing whole foods. Know that you are going through some tough stuff right now, and the important thing is to make an effort to take care of your body and soul with good clean food, peaceful surroundings, some type of movement, fresh air and sunshine and supportive people around you.

Comfort

IF YOU THINK of all the times in your life when you wanted some comfort food (bad day at work; long day with the kids; a heated argument with your best friend), most likely none of them hold a candle to the comfort you're seeking now. You have stupid, lonely, scary cancer and you feel like shit. You want to snuggle up and perhaps eat foods that remind you of your childhood, a warm summer's day or a cozy evening by the fireplace. So pass the mac 'n cheese, please. Or the ice cream. Or the hot cocoa. Or mashed potatoes and lots of gravy.

Okay, we get that. Heck, we lived that! We certainly aren't judging you. Just

Dirty Dozen

If you are prioritizing your produce pennies and need to know which fruits and veggies are most important to buy organic, we have the inside scoop here for you. Allow us to present the Dirty Dozen and the Clean Fifteen! Created by the Environmental Working Group, these two lists provide the lowdown on foods grown with the most and least amount of pesticides. Wash all produce well, use a scrub brush, and keep knives and cutting boards clean. If you want to take it a step further with conventional produce, especially during cancer treatment, you can also soak fruits and veggies in bit of white wine vinegar or food-grade hydrogen peroxide.

Visit www.ewg.org to download the lists as well as the app for your smart phone.

Dirty Dozen (buy these organic):

1. Apples
2. Celery
3. Sweet bell peppers
4. Peaches
5. Strawberries
6. Nectarines (imported)
7. Grapes
8. Spinach
9. Lettuce
10. Cucumbers
11. Blueberries (domestic)
12. Potatoes

Clean Fifteen (lowest in pesticides, so it's okay to buy conventional if you need to):

1. Onions
2. Corn (though often GMO)
3. Pineapples
4. Avocados
5. Cabbage
6. Sweet peas
7. Asparagus
8. Mangoes
9. Eggplant
10. Kiwi
11. Cantaloupe (domestic)
12. Sweet potatoes
13. Grapefruit
14. Watermelon
15. Mushrooms

remember that there may be another option that is just as comforting and is better for you. Looking for mac 'n cheese? Try our Squashy Macaroni and Cheeze (page 251). Want some cookies? It's really easy to whip up a quick batch of our No-Bake Oatmeal Raisin Balls (page 300). And if you really just want an afternoon of hiding under a mountain of blankets in bed with Ben and Jerry (hey, get your mind out of the gutter—we *do* mean the ice cream!) have your afternoon, then, but start nourishing your body again when dinnertime comes.

It's also important to look for comfort in other ways, besides food. Does putting on your pajamas and snuggling up on the couch with your favorite fleece blanket and a movie help you to relax? Perhaps you need some quality time with your sweetie or children. What about a hot bubble bath or a nap outside on your hammock? Food can be soothing, but we bet you can also find other ways to relax and find comfort.

In the Recipes

Comfort-food recipes include Banana Split Smoothie (page 202), Sweet Potato Fries with Peanut Dipping Sauce (page 240), Kale Pesto Linguini with Tomatoes (page 248), Roasted Buckwheat and Gravy (page 250), Squashy Macaroni and Cheeze (page 251), Move-Over Meatloaf (page 261), Key-Lime Custard Pie (page 299) and Pumpkin Loaf with Maple Glaze (page 304).

Surgery, Radiation, and Chemotherapy

EACH STAGE OF cancer treatment brings its own set of concerns and priorities, including the realm of food. Of course, you will want to chat with your doctor about your specific procedure and diagnosis and what, if any, restrictions you may have. But here are some general thoughts to keep in mind for various types of cancer-related treatments.

SURGERY: The body undergoes considerable stress and strain from anesthesia, and the surgical procedure itself creates significant trauma, so it's important to make sure you have as much nutritional support as possible both before and after surgery. That includes an increased amount of quality, plant-based protein to help your body recovery, heal and rebuild itself after the surgical procedure.

You may be asked to refrain from eating and drinking immediately prior to your surgery. But before that, keep your body well hydrated and fed. In the days following surgery, drinking plenty of fluids is helpful in flushing the anesthesia from your body and helps to get your digestive and excretory systems back up and running. Water is so important in recovery, so drink up!

Using arnica, a homeopathic remedy, can also be helpful in supporting healing from surgery. Begin with arnica two days prior to surgery and continue immediately afterwards (it is safe to take as soon as you wake up) for a week. It will help your body heal from trauma and bruising.

RADIATION: All of us are exposed to radiation on a daily basis. If you are also receiving radiation treatments you will want to speak with your radiation oncologist regarding your diet or wait until your treatments have ended to modify your diet. If you are looking to protect yourself from daily radiation exposure, having been exposed to radiation from X-rays and scans, or if you are recovering from radiation therapy, sea vegetables (see "Food Friends," in Chapter 3) and miso (fermented soy-bean paste) offer support for your body and have been used for generations in Asia. These foods may account for the lower cancer rates found in populations that consume a traditional Asian diet. Enjoy nori in sushi, kelp granules sprinkled on grains and veggies, kombu in your rice and beans and a daily bowl of miso soup. Miso soup can also help with the fatigue that often accompanies radiation treatment. Be sure you're also getting plenty of plant-based proteins to help your body with the healing it needs to do from radiation itself.

CHEMOTHERAPY: When undergoing chemo, sometimes food can be tough to figure out. Mouth sores and throat pain are common side effects of chemo that make eating quite difficult. These side effects can be incredibly frustrating, because you may be hungry, not feeling nauseous at all, and just can't eat much of anything because your mouth hurts. Ugh! You may discover that only certain foods, like citrus or tomatoes, aggravate mouth sores, or if your throat is really raw it may be that no solid food goes down easily. In these instances, stick with cool liquids like water and coconut water, and try some of our refreshment recipes without the citrus ingredients. Smoothies are perfect in this situation: You can add in plenty of filling, energizing food without having to be uncomfortable chewing and swallowing it. Soup may also be okay, but often heat will aggravate a raw mouth and throat, so be cautious with the soup's temperature.

———~~wwwww~~———

Your tastes for different foods may change, too. That special pasta dish you once loved may leave you feeling nauseous, or you may suddenly love to eat celery when before it was far too bland and boring for you. Especially in the days right after chemo, you may need to eat differently based on your changed tastes. Many people undergoing chemo experience what is often described as a metallic taste in their mouths, which makes everything taste funny and can leave you feeling nauseous. You may want food that is bland because too much flavor also triggers nausea (and be sure to drink plenty of water to help keep that nausea at bay), or you may want to enhance flavors and wake up those tired taste buds because you can't seem to really taste anything, or to get that darn metallic taste out of your mouth.

Just like with surgery and radiation, be sure to increase your protein intake when undergoing chemo. This will keep your energy and strength up and help to build and repair healthy cells in your body. When dealing with sores or "chemo mouth," try adding protein-rich foods to smoothies, like nut butters or hemp powder. Comfort food also becomes a necessity during chemo. You feel like crap and the idea of snuggling up in a cozy chair with your personal version of a comfort food seems just perfect. Do what you need to do to get through this time.

When going through cancer treatment, the side effects can be grueling or, for some, they may not be too extreme. Every person is affected differently. Getting the right foods into your body can make a huge difference in how your body is able to cope with side effects and how quickly you recover. We felt the difference during our treatments when we changed our diets, and we know you can, too! Our advice? In a nutshell: Drink plenty of fluids, especially water. Eat nutrient-dense foods whenever you can get them down. Try to find "upgraded" alternatives to the not-so-healthy stuff you might be craving. Use our notes in the Recipes section as well as information in this chapter to help you navigate the best foods for dealing with certain side effects. And above all else, know that what you eat really can make a difference.

CHAPTER 8

It's Okay to
Eat Chocolate and Cry

We are here to help you do all you can to prevent and kick cancer, but your Girlfriends also realize that some days you may want to crawl under the covers and wish it would all just go away. We know. We've been there. And we are here to tell you, it is okay to eat chocolate and cry! (Just make sure it's dark chocolate!) When you're feeding your body delicious cancer-fighting food and getting the support you need, you might be feeling like you are thriving, not just surviving. But you may also have times when, despite your best intentions, you are feeling really blue and a green vegetable doesn't pass your lips for a couple days. All is not lost! If you "screw up" (whatever that means!), it doesn't mean all hope is gone. It's okay: Get back up on the Cancer-Kicking Wagon and keep on going!

Keeping Up Appearances

EVERY CANCER WARRIOR has days when she is feeling worn out. Maybe you don't feel like a warrior at all. Maybe on top of dealing with cancer, you are beating yourself up for feeling down, depressed and angry. Just like we covered in Chapter 2, you don't need to define yourself as the Cancer Warrior, the Cancer Survivor or even the Cancer Misfit! You don't always need to be strong or optimistic, or put on a happy face for the people around you.

We know how hard it can be once you believe you have your cancer "image" established. Your girlfriends are sending you the Wonder Woman T-shirts and telling you how amazing you are. While this is all important and keeps the cancer-fighting

Annette:

Sometimes it can go the other way, too. I got to a space during treatment when I made peace with my situation and decided to enjoy each day as best as I could. I actually got asked by a friend, expecting me to be down and out, if I was in denial about my situation! Guess she didn't understand how I could have cancer *and* a smile on my face!

fires stoked, you may feel like you can't show your sadness, your weakness or your fear. You don't want to admit that you spent the day yelling at your family, or curled up in a ball on the couch watching *Sex and the City* reruns instead of blogging as Miss Inspirational about your life-changing cancer journey. Drop the pressure. Does it mean you are not awesome and strong and inspirational? Heck, no. Get real with yourself. And try getting real with those around you. Take a leap, and let them in.

What's more, sometimes it feels as if we, on top of dealing with our cancer stuff, need to take care of the fears, emotions and concerns of those around us. We find ourselves comforting the very people who should be there comforting us, acting strong in moments in which we actually don't feel that way. Don't add this to your cancer "to do" list! As we chatted about in the "Stupid Lonely Cancer" section in Chapter 2, though it can sometimes be difficult for those around us, you are not responsible at this moment (well, *ever*, really!) for their well-being. This is about you and getting the care and support you need. While appreciating and showing love to those around us, we serve ourselves and our loved ones best when we let them know what is going on with us and what we need, rather than putting on a warrior face when we're feeling anything but fierce.

This is also a good time to find and call on some cancer peeps. There is nothing like talking to an understanding girlfriend who has been where you are now and who really "gets" what is going on with you. And if you aren't up for talking about the cancer roller-coaster with anyone, find a trusty journal to share all your thoughts, feelings, ups and downs with. Sometimes when it all felt like it was too much for us, we would just pick up our journals and write, write, write—a continual stream-of-consciousness flow—until we felt a pleasant exhaustion, an emotional purge of sorts. Just know you are not alone with all of this, and even though it may not seem like it right now, nothing—not even the worst moments of cancer crap—lasts forever.

Be Bad

~~~~~~~~~~~~~

WITH SO MUCH on the line with a cancer diagnosis—we are thrown into life versus death mode—we may try even harder than ever to be "perfect," and that just creates a whole lot more of one thing: stress. So much of our life and our cancer treatment is focused on being "good," on getting to our appointments, managing work and home life (or arranging for someone else to do so), eating the right food and exercising. While this is super important, it can leave us not only exhausted but constantly feeling like we aren't quite "good" enough.

For some of us, we've become masterful self-critics. Whatever it is, we are somehow "not (fill in the blank) enough." But whose rules and beliefs are we living by? And is possibly paying the price of these judgments with our health acceptable? Just humor your Girlfriends and ponder these questions as you travel along your cancer journey.

Humans, including cancer chicks, aren't perfect and we shouldn't pretend to be. Pretending to be perfect is actually an inauthentic way to live life, and we are all about getting real here. So step into your integrity and embrace your "bad" side. Try being "bad" for a day, or even part of a day. What does that mean exactly? It means

Down and Out

Cancer can be a time for change and growth. For many of us, it can also sometimes be a time for feelings of helplessness and despair. Sinking into sadness for a while is natural. But if your depression lingers, you may want to seek help from a doctor or therapist, preferably someone with specialized training and experience in working with individuals facing cancer. Don't be afraid to ask for help: We lose valuable energy needed for kicking cancer when we keep things looking as if they are okay when they are not.

Delving into some of the self-care practices we've introduced in this chapter is really important when you are feeling down in the dumps. Receiving healing touch, sitting in silence or getting outside to move and feel the sun shine on your face can lift spirits and bring some peace. And we promise that eating real food, as we introduce in this book, will help you feel better and stronger emotionally and psychologically.

Make sure you get the support you need to make your self-care a priority, including your food. Have a girlfriend or partner enjoy some self-care with you (they need it too!), or ask them to keep you accountable for scheduling it for yourself. For most cancer chicks, feelings of depression last for a short time, and acknowledging them and realizing such feelings are normal help us to move on to the next phase.

doing something that you don't feel you should do. Want to skip writing thank-you notes? Want to thumb your nose at hanging out with certain friends or family members? Want to chow down on some less-than-healthy food? Go ahead: do it! We are not encouraging a "let all hell break loose" attitude 24/7. What we want to

Kendall:

I didn't intentionally try to be "bad" during my cancer stuff, but I didn't restrict myself either. I did what felt good to me. I lived in the moment. If that meant eating a slice of chocolate cake one day, then that was fine. If it meant not cleaning my house for a week because I was too tired, great! I think my first experience in being "bad" was right after my surgery in the hospital. So many wonderful friends and family wanted to visit, and I had a room full of them immediately following the surgery. It was way too much. I was exhausted and vomiting just from trying to give everyone a chance to be there and see that I was okay. I actually tried to be a hostess, when I could hardly move and was in constant pain. After that, my husband and I decided to turn down any requests for visits so I could recuperate as I needed to, and it was one of the best decisions we made. Sometimes being "bad" just means not trying to please everyone else and doing exactly what *you* want or need. Even if that means saying no.

encourage you to do is give yourself permission to not have to be perfect.

This is also an opportunity to question and look deeply to see if you have the "disease to please." If, perhaps unknowingly, you have given away your personal power to other people, to life situations, or to unquestioned belief systems, cancer can offer an opportunity to reclaim the privilege and responsibility of being in charge of your own life and of learning what it means to please yourself.

This is all stuff that you may not want to hear or face right now. Isn't dealing with the cancer hard enough as it is? But let us assure you that if you can shift your perspective to one of seeing how this disease is asking you to grow and change, then having been hit with a diagnosis can also turn into an opportunity to learn, reclaim lost or forgotten aspects of yourself and strengthen your voice and, ultimately, your life.

Start a Love Affair

———~~~~~———

AND WHILE WE'RE on the topic of being bad: The cancer journey is the perfect time to start a love affair. A love affair with yourself, that is. While a cancer diagnosis shows us quite clearly that in the end we stand alone—it is our bodies that receive the treatment and we ourselves who are called on to grapple with the notions of life and death—it also shows us that we are the only ones who can complete ourselves and give ourselves the love and acceptance we want. Yep, that's right: No one else—not our family, our partners, our friends, anyone. We cannot control or manipulate others to give us the love we want, the way we want it, when and where we want it. But the good news is we *can* have it! How? We can give it to ourselves, by showing

Annette:

Something I pondered while going through the many surgeries necessary to deal with my cancers was: How much of me is left of me? How much of me was in that tissue or body part that was just removed? Can I still think of myself as whole? Can I feel whole? The surprising answer that came through to me was yes. In fact, as I shed my proverbial skin, I began to feel more whole, more "me" than I had before. How was that possible? While there were many things about cancer that seemed to rob me of much of my life, there was simultaneously something about it that woke me up out of my daily stupor and brought me fully into my being. Something that showed me that what makes Annette *Annette* isn't my hair or my breasts or anything of that nature. By force, it taught me that I am far more than any of my body parts and that they do not make me who I am.

up and being present with and for ourselves in a loving, completely accepting way. Sound pretty radical? It is!

So what happens when instead of loving ourselves we go looking "out there" for the fulfillment of all our desires and wishes? Well, for one, it makes us painfully dependent on the actions of others and on situations over which we have no control. And it also leaves literally "no one home" with us! We've left ourselves, and are trying to get from other people and situations the love we already have and are. No wonder we feel all alone! We aren't even there with and for ourselves. Making the promise to unconditionally love and be present for ourselves sounds simple, and for some of us, it is. Others benefit from the guidance of a therapist or another supportive individual. Whatever it takes, find what is helpful for you and spend time working on developing complete love for and acceptance of yourself.

On a similar note, it can be particularly hard to embrace and appreciate our bodies now. Some cancer girlfriends feel betrayed by their bodies for developing cancer. Others can't accept the altered landscape of their physique that often follows cancer treatment. From new surgery scars and hair loss, to hot flashes and lost libidos, is there anything still to love about this body? Absolutely! Our body is there for us, moment by moment, heartbeat after heartbeat, doing its very best and offering us a gift we often don't take the time to be aware of and appreciate. Do your best to live life with this realization: "Yeah, here is my issue, here's my stuff . . . but I'm not broken. I am a *whole* human being who has cancer [or who had cancer; or is concerned about cancer]." Honor your body by making the commitment to love and express gratitude for it.

Another fantastic way to show yourself some love and be sure you are taking time to actually do the things you love is by creating a Loving Me List. In your Loving Me List, you can include everything that makes you happy and truly lights you up inside. Do you have a blast getting in the kitchen and baking with a friend? Does tak-

Vitamin D

There's been much excitement in recent years about the role that vitamin D plays in the creation and functioning of healthy cells in the body. Vitamin D not only protects our bones and boosts our immune system, it has been shown to block the growth of cancer tumors. Studies have suggested that people with higher vitamin D levels at the time of cancer diagnosis often have a higher survival rate, and also suggest that increasing vitamin D levels after cancer diagnosis may improve chances of survival.

Ask your physician for a blood test to check your levels—the script should request a test for vitamin D 25-OH D—and make sure your levels are optimal. If not, you may require supplementation and also want to engage in some short, safe sunshine bathing to boost this anti-cancer hormone.

ing a walk on the beach and smelling the ocean make you feel fresh and alive? Does treating yourself to a pedicure relax you and make you feel pretty and pampered? Add it to your list! Here's an example of a Loving Me List with some things that bring us happiness. Feel free to steal some of our ideas for your own list!

- Getting together with girlfriends for dinner
- Hiking when fall foliage is at its peak
- Picking wild raspberries and blackberries
- Yoga
- Foot soaks with essential oils
- Working in the flower garden

- Curling up with a blanket, hot tea and a favorite book
- Collecting sea shells on the beach
- Shopping for and finding a fabulous new pair of shoes (on sale!)

Chow Down on Chocolate

AND SPEAKING OF love affairs, did someone mention chocolate? Hello, my love!

We have all heard of the antioxidant benefits found in chocolate. Antioxidants are substances that reduce ongoing cellular damage caused by oxidative reactions. You may also have heard of a type of antioxidant called polyphenols. These are protective chemicals found in plant foods such as red wine and green tea. Chocolate is particularly rich in polyphenols. Why then has chocolate gotten such a bad rap? It's the ingredients we add to it: Most chocolate on the market today is highly processed, contains milk and is loaded with refined sweeteners that dangerously raise blood sugar and cholesterol levels. What to do? Ditch the Snickers Bar, and get some good-quality dark chocolate: The higher the cacao content, the better it is for you. Want to kick it even harder? Look for raw chocolate, a whole food with lots of healthy goodness.

Kendall:

Some of the recipes in the cookbook section use raw cacao. It's amazing and so much better for you than any other chocolate you can buy. And cacao not only tastes amazing, it is anticancer as well! Yes, it's a healthy food! Plus, because it's so decadent and satisfying, you really don't need to eat much to be choco-happy. So go ahead and give it a try (like you need any convincing).

Need some more reasons to eat chocolate?!

- Contains theobromine, a milder stimulant than caffeine

- Increases energy

- Supports the immune system

- Strengthens the cardiovascular system

- Stimulates neurotransmitters in your brain (such as serotonin) to help reduce depression and to give a sense of euphoria or a sense of well-being

- One of the highest dietary sources of magnesium, a vital mineral for healthy cell function

- A good source of iron and calcium

- Considered to be a mild aphrodisiac (*bow chicka bow wow!*)

Self-Care XOXO

——◦◦◦◦◦◦◦◦——

SO OFTEN WE go through life running from one thing to the next. We are busy with work and family responsibilities, putting the needs of partners, children, friends and bosses above our own. We believe we don't have the time to take care of ourselves, whether it is moving our bodies with exercise, preparing and eating healthy food, finding moments of balance and stillness in our days or even taking a deep breath and appreciating our bodies for all they does for us day after day, month after month, year after year.

For many of us, a cancer diagnosis is a wakeup call in a number of ways. We have said ourselves, and have heard many of our cancer peeps say, "I knew I was burning the candle at both ends. I knew I was stressed and wasn't taking care of myself," when speaking of the time prior to getting hit with the Big C news. Suddenly a diagnosis puts everything into glaring perspective. Now it's just not about having low energy, flabby abs or edgy nerves. It is about surviving, and the stakes are high.

If you are serious about getting healthy, then now is a good time to get serious with self-care. Your amazing body is busy kicking cancer, so show it some love! Here's the low-down on some of our self-care faves:

Reiki

Reiki (pronounced RAY-key) is a Japanese word representing universal life energy, the energy that is all around us. Reiki is both this vital life-force energy and also the technique used to access that energy to balance and energize yourself (you can learn to give Reiki to yourself) or others on physical, emotional, mental and spiritual levels. A Reiki practitioner places her hands usually above, sometimes on, the recipient and amplifies and channels universal life-force energy through herself to the person receiving the Reiki. Reiki energy has several basic effects: It can bring about deep relaxation, eliminate energy blockages and has been said to help speed the body's ability to heal itself and to relieve tension and pain.

Annette:

When I was going through chemotherapy, a Reiki practitioner volunteered in my cancer center to give Reiki to individuals on chemo days. Ask if your hospital has a similar offering or contact a Reiki practitioner to see if they are willing to work on a sliding scale with individuals undergoing treatment for cancer.

Reflexology

Reflexology is the practice of applying pressure to the feet and hands utilizing specific thumb, finger and hand techniques. It is based on a system of zones and reflex areas that reflect an image of the body on the feet and hands with a premise that such work effects a physical change in the body. Studies have shown reflexology to ease symptoms of pain, nausea and anxiety for those undergoing chemotherapy. One of the main benefits of reflexology is a reduction in stress levels. And let's face it: What's not to love about getting your tootsies some TLC!

Yoga

If you think you need to be able to bend yourself into a pretzel to do yoga, think again. And if you think there is no way you can do yoga while kicking cancer, think again, too. Our bodies can heal and strengthen faster when we are able to slow down and loosen some of the tightness we tend to carry with us. While acute stress has its place in our biology, chronic stress leads to chronic tension, both in the body and the mind. And worse, it actually depresses the function of the immune system and those natural killer cells so important in giving cancer cells the boot. Yoga offers the opportunity to stretch our bodies, breathe deeply and relieve stress that has been shown to promote the growth of tumors. There are different branches of yoga, so you can find a style that best suits you. Make sure to discuss with your instructor any restrictions you have due to surgery or other treatment, and go at your own pace.

Bach flowers

Bach Flower tinctures are a safe and natural method of emotional healing. Based on homeopathic principles, they gently restore the balance between mind and body by helping to eliminate negative emotions, such as, fear, worry, anger and indecision that cause stress and imbalance. You choose the appropriate tincture for your emotional concern and add several drops to your drink or place directly under your tongue.

Meditation

In our lives we are normally so busy doing and thinking that it can seem incredibly challenging to just sit and "be." We are so convinced we have to "do something" and as we are constantly trying to do, we constrict space and constrict our bodies. Meditation is a way of releasing constriction and creating spaciousness in our bodies, our minds and our thoughts. Into this spaciousness often comes intuition, answers and insights.

There are many ways in which to practice meditation. One of the simplest methods, and one that is always available no matter where we are, is focusing attention on the breath. Since breathing is automatic, placing attention on your inhalations and exhalations can enable you to more easily drop into a place of *observing thoughts and feelings without attachment*. Leaving our usual habit of blindly following all of our thoughts (which has often been referred to as "monkey mind" attention: hopping here and there and everywhere), meditation offers your attention the opportunity to be neutral and focused on a constant: the breath (or a mantra, or a candle, for example).

Getting Quiet

Here's a quick and easy introduction to sitting meditation:

1. Arrange yourself comfortably in an upright sitting posture, one in which your body breathes freely.

2. Give yourself permission to simply rest, settle in and allow your breathing to find its own natural rhythm.

3. Gather your attention and place it on the rhythmic movement of your body that is created by your breathing.

4. Don't try to stop the thoughts that arise, and they will—but when you notice you are paying attention to the inner dialogue and stories that distract you, simply bring your attention back and refocus on the movement of your body.

5. (optional) You can start with just 5 or 10 minutes once a day and build slowly to 15 or 20 minutes. If you resonate with meditation practice it could benefit you to look for a local instructor.

Provided by Gabriel Rocco, mind-body health specialist and contemplative counselor, www.contemplative-arts.com

In this state of stable, nonjudgmental focus, awareness is drawn inward to its essence and we can experience moments of peace and ease. Meditation can be practiced on your own or in a group. When beginning to meditate, it can be helpful to receive some instruction and have the support of a community of others engaged in the practice. For us, the realization that we didn't have to be blind slaves to our automatic thinking, and its sometimes frightening stories, brought about a complete change of perspective and understanding. Getting our time in on the meditation cushion becomes a happy necessity, an oasis in the cancer whirlwind, which sends out ripples of a "peace that passes all understanding" throughout our days.

Dancing in the living room

Put on your favorite tracks and just move to the music. Maybe it is gentle and slow or rockin' and jumpin'. Allow your body to find its rhythm and enjoy your own personal disco. Or sing your heart out *American Idol*-style to whatever song matches your mood. Both can have a cleansing, strengthening effect and a chance to turn off your thoughts and just groove!

Walks, sunshine and vitamin D

Hanging out on the couch all day is sometimes inevitable when you are going through the cancer crap. The thought of moving your body can make you cringe in anticipation of the pain. (Although sometimes once you get gently moving, the pain actually lessens as your body warms up and releases tension.) When you do have a day that you are able to get up and move a bit, try a gentle walk. If you are feeling really weak,

Kendall:

Before my big surgery, my husband helped me create a special sanctuary outdoors where I would be able to relax, heal and take in the fresh air and sunshine. We had a little gazebo that we turned into what we later called my "zen palace." We added comfy chairs and my very own cushy lounge chair, some plants, a small, inexpensive fountain, an electric fan for the really hot days and some little chains of lights for the evening. I spent a lot of time in there, snoozing, reading, relaxing or chatting with family and friends. I truly believe that my little zen palace helped me to heal, balance and find peace during the times I needed it most.

make sure you take along a buddy. Sometimes just a short walk, and the chance to soak up some sunshine and make some vitamin D, can lift your spirits and give you a boost. And if you're not up to walking, find a comfy chair and spend some time outside in the fresh air catching a few rays.

Cooking Up Love

- Taking the time to learn about real good-for-you food
- Realizing that your meal is not just there to fill a hole in your stomach, but rather to nourish and support your body
- Making the connection between what you eat and how you feel

WHEN THESE SHIFTS occur in your mind and your life, you are stepping up to the plate (literally) to take care of yourself and your life. When you dice, chop, sauté and steam, you are practicing radical self-care and self-love: You're not just making dinner, you are caring for your body and your life!

Believe it or not, eating plant-based whole foods cooked with love helped both of us combat sadness and anxiety when dealing with cancer. To our own amazement and the amazement of everyone around us, we started feeling better, looking brighter and enjoying life more than we ever had before—while in cancer treatment! There really is something to eating your veggies, chewing your grains and making space in your mind.

Just remember that healthy self-care and lifestyle habits done from a place of obligation, fear, self-judgment and a less-than-whole mentality create stress and nix the juicy benefits. Practice them out of love and appreciation for yourself, your body, your life. Use them not to "fix" yourself but to care for and support yourself whether you are trying to prevent cancer or recover from it.

Life After Cancer—Now What?

When people finish active treatment for cancer, they are sometimes disappointed that life after cancer doesn't feel as good as expected. Or they may be asking, "Now what?" and find themselves wondering where to start with rebuilding their lives. After I finished cancer treatment, I found that there was this "emotional aftermath"—I expected to be happy again but found myself experiencing a rollercoaster of emotions.

It's important to realize that if you're someone who has similar challenges, you're not alone. It's very common in cancer survivors. Emotional recovery from cancer is a process that takes time, but there are things we can do to help the healing process along. The time and effort it takes to heal the emotional impact from cancer is worthwhile because you will be able to move forward more easily in your life.

Be gentle to yourself throughout this recovery process. Some people, myself included, have thought that at one time or another they were "going crazy" or that something is "wrong with me" because they're feeling strong emotions after treatment is over. It's important to remind yourself that you're **NOT** going crazy and there's **NOTHING** wrong with you: You're just experiencing the emotional recovery process, and it takes time.

One crucial way to help with the issues that come up after finishing cancer treatment is to get support in whatever way works for you. There are support groups and one-on-one peer support programs for cancer survivors (in-person and online) where confidentiality is highly valued. When I was recovering from cancer, I found my counselor to be the best type of support for me. She taught me skills and strategies that I still use to this day when I encounter difficult times.

With support and persistence, it is possible to recover from the emotional impact of cancer and to reinvent your life with more meaning and purpose than ever before: A life you love. As Marilyn Monroe once said, "Sometimes good things fall apart so that better things can fall together." Provided by Dawn Pelletier Stratton, LCPC, Cancer Counselor, www.awakening.com

Group Hug!

~~~~~~~~~~~~

THANK YOU FOR taking us along on your cancer kicking journey. Whether you have cancer or are hoping to prevent it, we wrote this book for you, dear girl-friend, and we want you to know that we wish our words could jump off these pages and give you a big warm hug. You are amazing, and you are doing something wonderful for yourself just by reading this book and beginning to make changes in your diet and your life. We know you can do this. And don't worry - you're not alone! So let's get into the kitchen together and get cooking!

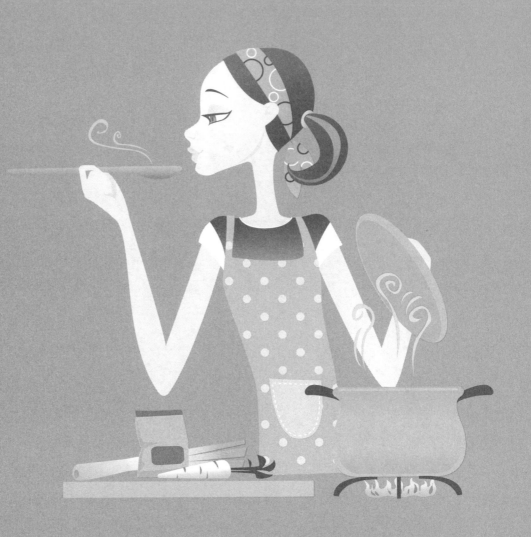

2

The Recipes

A Guide to Using the Recipes

Keep it Simple, Sister!

We can't wait for you to expand your world, get in the kitchen and start chowing down on some cancer-kicking food! We know you are going to love these super yummy recipes we used ourselves and are now sharing with you. But listen to your Girlfriends: Don't stress! Of course, cooking and eating are about getting the best nutrition possible into your amazing body. Beyond that, it should also be about lightening up and having a bit of fun. So you've found a recipe that looks fantastic, but you're missing one of the ingredients? No worries—get creative and use what you've got. Being in the kitchen is a bit like being an artist: Let your creative juices out and go with the flow. Who knows? You may come up with your new favorite dish! Scared to try a new food? Don't be—you may end up loving it (and you'll benefit from all of the nutrient-rich goodness it provides). So have no fear: Dive in, explore and enjoy!

Kitchen Equipment

IN SEVERAL RECIPES we use some kitchen gear that you may want to have available in your cooking space. Some are a necessity; others just make things easier for you. If you find you need to purchase most of these and are worried about the expense, just start with one or two and add more to your collection over time. Our favorites are the handheld immersion blender and food processor.

BLENDER—Blenders are also great for pureed soups and smoothies.

CHEF'S KNIFE—Keep this knife sharpened for some quick veggie chopping.

ELECTRIC JUICER—If you plan to do much juicing, you'll want a good juicer.

FOOD PROCESSOR—A food processor lessens the amount of work you need to do. Less chopping as well as an easy way to integrate a bunch of ingredients. Different attachments allow you to grate or slice foods in seconds.

GARLIC PRESS—A quick way to mince your garlic.

IMMERSION BLENDER—This is a handheld blender perfect for making pureed soups, smoothies and sauces.

MANDOLINE—This handheld tool makes slicing fruit and veggies a snap.

Recipe Benefits

FOR EACH RECIPE, you'll see we've listed the specific benefits directly under the recipe name, so you can focus on the recipes that can be helpful in dealing with your individual concerns. You can also see which are vegetarian, raw or vegan.

Here's a complete list of the benefits we spotlight:

Blood Boosting	Immune Boosting
Brain Boosting	Mouth Sore Friendly
Comfort Food	Mood Balancing
Constipation Kicking	Nausea Nixing
Dehydration Defending	Raw
Detoxifying	Respiratory-System Support
Fatigue Fighting and Adrenal Support	Vegan
Hormone Balancing	Vegetarian

A Note About Yields

We're providing you with the actual recipe yield versus number of servings. This is because serving sizes can vary from person to person and don't take individual needs and preferences into account.

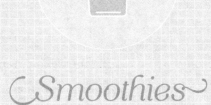

Smoothies

Oatmeal-Carrot Cookie Smoothie

comfort food | fatigue fighting and adrenal support | mood balancing |
raw | vegan | vegetarian

This is a delicious smoothie that makes you feel like you're having a dessert, but everything in it is super good for you! Rolled oats help you get in some energy-sustaining whole grains. Carrot offers vitamin A and C and because it's a root veggie, it helps bring you some grounding energy (so drink it up when you're feeling a little ditsy!). Banana sweetens and cinnamon and ginger are yummy cancer-fighting spices that complete this tasty treat. Enjoy as a mid-afternoon pick-me-up!

Yield: makes 18 ounces

1 large carrot, roughly chopped

3 tablespoons rolled oats

1 cup Almond Mylk (page 318) or store-bought

1 large banana

1 tablespoon ground flax seeds

3 large ice cubes

½ teaspoon pure vanilla extract

½ teaspoon ground cinnamon

¼ teaspoon ground ginger

¼ teaspoon ground nutmeg

2 teaspoons dried coconut, shredded and unsweetened

For less powerful blenders, grate the carrot. Add all ingredients except coconut to a blender and blend for one minute or until mostly smooth. Pour into individual glasses and sprinkle shredded coconut on top.

Kendall's Tasty Tip: If you like your smoothie a little thicker, try adding more ice or use a frozen banana.

Chocolate Malt Smoothie

comfort food | fatigue fighting and adrenal support |
raw | vegan | vegetarian

Remember when we talked about comfort foods? This smoothie is definitely one of them. It tastes just like chocolate malt, but with magnesium-rich raw cacao, no dairy and no refined sugars. Maca helps give it that malty flavor and pineapple and dates sweeten. This smoothie is soothing on the mouth and throat during chemo and has plenty of protein from the hemp seeds. As an added bonus, maca provides stamina and helps balance hormones.

Yield: makes about 20 ounces

1 vanilla bean

1½ cups of nondairy milk
(like soy, almond or hemp)

⅓ cup frozen pineapple cubes

¼ cup hemp seeds

¼ cup unrefined coconut oil, melted

3 tablespoons raw cacao powder

1 tablespoon maca

3 Medjool dates, pits removed

4 ice cubes

Slice open the vanilla bean pod and scrape out contents by sliding the tip of a sharp knife down the middle of the inside of the bean. Add all ingredients to a blender and mix at low speed for one minute, then medium speed for another minute until smooth. For thinner consistency, add extra non-dairy milk or water.

Annette's Tasty Tip: This is a definite comfort food for me. It reminds me of the milkshakes I had as a kid, but this one has many more health-promoting ingredients in it.

Tropical Island Smoothie

immune boosting | mood balancing | raw | vegan | vegetarian

We want to take you away to the islands, so stick your toes in the sand, grab a glass of this sweet concoction and let the stress melt away. Mango is rich in polyphenolic flavonoid antioxidant compounds and has been found to protect against leukemia and colon and breast cancers. Pineapple is rich in vitamin C, an antioxidant that helps protect the body from harmful free radicals. So while you're pretending you're on the beach (or maybe you really are—hey, pack a cooler with your yummy smoothie!), know your body is getting some cancer-fighting goodies.

Yield: makes 16 ounces

¼ cup Almond Mylk (page 318) or store-bought

½ cup coconut water

1 banana

1 cup frozen mango pieces

½ cup fresh or frozen pineapple

½ cup fresh strawberries

2 tablespoons dried coconut, shredded and unsweetened

3 ice cubes

Add all ingredients to a blender and mix for one minute, or until mostly smooth. If a thinner smoothie is desired, add more coconut water or Almond Mylk and blend for a few more seconds.

Annette's Tasty Tip: Decorate your smoothie with a slice a pineapple or even one of those cute little umbrellas. Presenting our food in a fun and interesting way helps us enjoy it even more and adds an extra dose of happiness and love.

Gorgeous Green Smoothie

blood boosting | brain boosting | dehydration defending | detoxifying | fatigue fighting and adrenal support | immune boosting | mood balancing | raw | vegan | vegetarian

We've talked about how important it is to get those leafy greens into your diet. Adding them to a smoothie is a super easy way to get your green on and nourish your blood and immune system. Adding fruit with soluble fiber makes the smoothie creamy and more palatable. Plus, this smoothie only calls for four ingredients and a few ice cubes: easy!

Yield: makes 16 ounces

2 cups nondairy milk (like soy, almond or hemp)

1 cup packed kale leaves, stemmed

1 banana

½ avocado, pit removed

3 ice cubes

Add all ingredients to a blender and blend for one minute or until smooth.

Kendall's Tasty Tip: To make this smoothie a little heftier and more satiating, try adding two tablespoons of a raw nut butter of your choice.

Mint Chocolate-Chip Smoothie

comfort food | fatigue fighting and adrenal support | immune boosting |
mood balancing | vegetarian

This smoothie reminds us of mint chocolate-chip milkshakes, and it's good enough to have for dessert! Instead of chocolate chips, we use cacao nibs, small pieces of the raw cacao bean. They can be found at most health-food stores and are an excellent source of magnesium.

Yield: makes 20 ounces

1 frozen large banana, very ripe

1 tablespoon cacao nibs

10 drops pure peppermint extract

1½ cups coconut milk

½ cup baby spinach, packed

1 tablespoon raw cacao powder

1 tablespoon real maple syrup or honey

3-4 mint leaves, optional, plus a sprig for garnish

Add all ingredients to a blender and mix at low speed for thirty seconds, then medium speed for another minute until smooth. Add mint leaves if desired and blend for a few more seconds. Pour into a glass and garnish with a sprig of mint leaves.

Kendall's Tasty Tip: Raw cacao nibs and powder offer the health benefits of raw food. And you can read about all of the cancer-kicking and mood-boosting benefits of cacao in Chapter 8, "It's Okay to Eat Chocolate and Cry."

Superfood Smoothie

blood boosting | detoxifying | fatigue fighting and adrenal support | immune boosting |
mouth sore friendly | raw | vegan | vegetarian

This smoothie has some superfood ingredients that you won't find in most grocery store chains, so you will need to visit a health-food store. Hemp powder is made from hemp seeds and is full of protein and magnesium. Maca we've mentioned as being a hormone balancer, and dulse is a nutrient-rich sea veggie that you can find in small flakes in a shaker or bag at the health-food store. Avocados provide many essential nutrients including B vitamins, vitamin E, potassium and folic acid. Add a little sweet fruit and you've got one kickin' smoothie!

Yield: makes 20 ounces

8 ounces Almond Mylk (page 318) or store-bought

2 ice cubes

½ avocado, pit removed

½ banana

½ cup blueberries

½ fresh mango, extra ripe, chopped

1 kale leaf, stem removed

1½ tablespoons hemp powder

½ teaspoon raw maca powder

½ tablespoon goji berry powder

½ teaspoon teaspoon dulse sea vegetable flakes

½ tablespoon honey

Combine all ingredients in a blender and mix at medium speed for about one minute until mostly smooth. If a thinner smoothie is desired, add more water or almond milk and blend for a few more seconds.

Annette's Tasty Tip: If you aren't able to find some of these superfoods like maca, hemp and goji powder at your local health-food store, try going online to NavitasNaturals.com to order them. Find dulse sea vegetable flakes in a shaker in the Asian section of your grocery or health-food store.

Berry Almond Smoothie

brain boosting | constipation kicking | dehydration defending | fatigue fighting and adrenal support | immune boosting | mood balancing | mouth sore friendly | raw | vegan | vegetarian

This smoothie is energizing, filling and super tasty! Bananas offer potassium to help replenish lost electrolytes, and berries give a boost of antioxidants, those awesome little cancer fighters. You get your protein and some fabulous nutrients, like iron, calcium and magnesium from the almonds. Anemia is common for those undergoing chemotherapy treatment and in many other people, and iron can help to treat this. Almonds are also helpful in relieving constipation.

Yield: makes 24 ounces

12 ounces Almond Mylk (page 318) or store-bought

1 banana

½ cup fresh or frozen raspberries

½ cup fresh or frozen strawberries

3 tablespoons raw almond butter

Combine all ingredients in a blender and mix at medium speed for about one minute or until mostly smooth. If a thinner smoothie is desired, add more water or almond milk and blend for a few more seconds.

Kendall's Tasty Tip: Smoothies were my go-to food during chemotherapy when I was too tired to spend time making meals and I wanted something to fill me up.

Banana Split Smoothie

comfort food | dehydration defending | mood balancing | mouth sore friendly | nausea nixing | vegan | vegetarian

If you grew up like we did associating a trip to the Dairy Queen with summer, special treats and love, you might find yourself craving that feeling from time to time. If you want to enjoy the memories and the taste without all the unhealthy ingredients, try this recipe. It's a banana split you can drink and it's good for you—need we say more? Well, we'll add that if you can't find a vanilla bean, go ahead and add one teaspoon of pure vanilla extract.

Yield: makes 16 ounces

1 vanilla bean, split lengthwise, insides scraped

¾ cup Almond Mylk (page 318) or store-bought

¾ cup coconut milk*

1 banana

½ cup frozen strawberries

1 tablespoon raw cacao powder

1 tablespoon honey or brown-rice syrup

Add all ingredients to a blender and mix at low speed for one minute, then medium speed for another minute until mostly smooth. If a thinner smoothie is desired, add more almond milk and blend for a few more seconds.

Annette's Tasty Tip: For a frothy consistency, use frozen bananas. We like to keep a bag of frozen banana pieces in our freezer for just such an occasion as this.

*Coconut milk from a can may separate (the milk and cream separate when stored). Whisk together before measuring.

Super Berry Booster Smoothie

brain boosting | dehydration defending | immune boosting | raw | vegan | vegetarian

Berries are loaded with antioxidants and are amazing little cancer fighters. Add in some superfood berries like goji and açai and you get one delicious and nutrient-rich concoction. Açai contains essential amino acids and polyunsaturated and monounsaturated fatty acids, which are essential to human health and may help reduce cancer risk. Goji berries are rich in vitamins B1, B2 and B6 and are known to be powerful immune boosters.

Yield: makes 24 ounces

1 cup fresh or frozen berries (raspberry, blueberry, strawberry, cranberry, blackberry)

12 ounces water

1 tablespoon açai powder

1 tablespoon goji powder

Ice cubes

Mint leaves

Add the first four ingredients to a blender and mix at low speed for thirty seconds, then medium speed for another minute until smooth. Add ice for desired consistency and blend again. Pour into glasses and garnish with sprigs of mint leaves.

Kendall's Tasty Tip: Frozen berries can also be used with little or no ice. I love to go berry picking and freeze berries to use during the off-season. If you can pick your own, that's even better and puts some local love into your smoothie! Find the superfood berries and powders in health-food-stores or online, but if you can't find them, just using a combination of other berries is very health promoting!

Protein Powerhouse Smoothie

blood boosting | dehydration defending | detoxifying | fatigue fighting and adrenal support |
immune boosting | mouth sore friendly | vegetarian

If you're feeling tired and weak, which is a common side effect of cancer treatment, you may need to up your protein intake. This protein-packed smoothie is loaded with foods that will help keep your energy up during chemo, radiation, after surgery or any time you may need that extra boost.

Yield: makes 24 ounces

1 tablespoon flax seeds

2 cups Sunny Hemp Mylk (page 316) or store-bought

¼ cup raw cashews

½ avocado, pit removed

1 banana

1 tablespoon spirulina powder

1 tablespoon honey

3 ice cubes

Grind flax seeds in blender or coffee-bean grinder. Add all ingredients to a blender and mix at low speed for thirty seconds, then medium speed for another minute until smooth.

Annette's Tasty Tip: Spirulina is a micro saltwater plant that is three to four times higher in protein than beef or fish. It can be purchased in powder form in health-food stores and is a wonderful addition to a plant-based diet for the protein, B vitamins and minerals phosphorus, calcium, magnesium and iron.

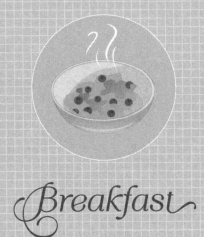

Breakfast

Simple Cinnamon Kasha

comfort food | fatigue fighting and adrenal support |
nausea nixing | vegan | vegetarian

Sometimes the best meals are the simplest ones. This is a snuggle-up-on-the-couch, in-your-pajamas breakfast that will fill you up and warm you up. It was an easy go-to meal during our chemo days when we needed a satisfying breakfast that provided some comfort at the same time. Kasha is a porridge made from whole buckwheat groats that have been roasted, creating a strong, somewhat nutty flavor. It's also gluten-free, despite "wheat" in its name, and is actually part of the rhubarb family.

Yield: makes 2 cups

1 cup kasha (roasted buckwheat)

1 teaspoon ground cinnamon

¼ cup Almond Mylk (page 318) or store-bought

Cook the kasha according to the grains cooking chart on page 244. Stir in the cinnamon and Almond Mylk and serve.

Eggless Broccoli-Tomato Frittata

comfort food | fatigue fighting and adrenal support | hormone balancing |
immune boosting | vegan | vegetarian

This flavorful breakfast dish is so delicious and really fills you up. It's always a big hit whenever we share it with family and friends, and they usually don't realize it's made with tofu instead of eggs until we tell them. This keeps in the fridge for a couple of days and goes well with a scoop of quinoa or some sautéed greens like the Garlic Lover's Kale (page 226).

Yield: makes 8 slices

1 small onion, diced

1 small head broccoli, chopped (1 cup)

2 tablespoons olive oil

2 cloves garlic, finely chopped

1 medium tomato, diced

⅓ cup fresh parsley, packed, chopped

6 medium mushrooms, chopped

1 package firm tofu (14 ounces)

¼ cup unsweetened rice milk

4 teaspoons arrowroot or cornstarch

2 heaping tablespoons nutritional yeast

¼ teaspoon paprika

1 teaspoon Dijon mustard

½ teaspoon turmeric

1 teaspoon dried dill

1 teaspoon sea salt

⅛ teaspoon freshly ground black pepper

Preheat the oven to 375°F.

In a pan over medium heat, sauté the onion and broccoli in the olive oil for five minutes. Add the garlic, cover and cook for two more minutes. Add the tomato, parsley and mushrooms, and sauté for two minutes. Remove from heat and cover.

Place the tofu between two cutting boards or two plates and squeeze excess water out. In a food processor (or blender), combine the tofu, rice milk, cornstarch, nutritional yeast, paprika, mustard, tumeric, dill, salt and pepper. Process until smooth. This mixture can also be mixed well by hand in a large bowl if a food processor is not available. Scoop into a large bowl and stir in the sautéed vegetables. Pour into a pie plate or similar-sized baking dish. Bake for forty minutes. Remove from the oven and let stand five minutes before serving.

Kendall's Tasty Tip: My husband, who used to say tofu can never take the place of eggs, loves this dish. Use this recipe for your basic frittata and then try mixing it up with different veggies like asparagus, kale, spinach, leeks and bell peppers.

Tempeh Hash Over Collards

blood boosting | fatigue fighting and adrenal support | hormone balancing |
immune boosting | nausea nixing | vegan | vegetarian

This delicious tempeh hash is simple to make (just get someone to do the veggie chopping for you if you're healing from surgery, or use a food processor) and has many immune-boosting ingredients. Serving it over a nice dark leafy green, like collards, adds vital nutrients and will help give you an energy boost so you can get through your morning feeling whole and happy.

Yield: makes about 5 cups hash, 2½ cups collards

1 medium sweet potato
(2 cups, shredded)

2 medium gold potatoes
(2 cups, shredded)

1 package tempeh,
crumbled (8 ounces)

1 small yellow onion,
chopped (1 cup)

3 garlic cloves, finely chopped

6 white mushrooms, chopped

⅓ cup nutritional yeast

3 tablespoons fresh parsley,
chopped

½ teaspoon paprika

1 teaspoon sea salt

¼ teaspoon freshly ground
black pepper

2 tablespoons olive oil

2 bunches collard greens,
stems removed

Preheat the oven to 400°F.

Gently scrub the sweet and gold potatoes and manually grate or use a food processor. Combine the potatoes, tempeh, onion, garlic, mushrooms, yeast, parsley, paprika, salt and pepper in a bowl and stir in oil until well coated. Scoop the mixture onto two cookie sheets, creating a thin layer. Bake for thirty-five minutes, stirring once and paying particular attention to the corners, or until just beginning to brown on top.

While the tempeh hash is baking, prepare the collards: tightly roll the collards then cut cross-wise into thin ribbons (about ¼ inch). Add three tablespoons of water to a skillet and sauté the collards on medium-low heat for two to three minutes. Serve the tempeh hash over the collards.

Polenta with Warm Berry Compote

comfort food | fatigue fighting and adrenal support | immune boosting | vegetarian

Polenta is made from cornmeal, and there are usually two ways to buy cornmeal: steel-ground or stone-ground. Steel-ground retains fewer nutrients, as the husk and germ have been almost completely removed. Stone-ground preserves some of the germ and hull of the corn, so you end up with a more nutrient-rich grain. Stone-ground cornmeal should be stored in an airtight container in the refrigerator for up to three months. Steel-ground can stay in the pantry. You can also purchase polenta in three textures: coarse, medium and fine (corn flour). Experiment with all three to decide which you like best for the polenta.

Yield: makes 4 cups cornmeal, about 2 cups compote

Compote:

1 tablespoon unrefined coconut oil

Juice from one small orange (or ¼ cup orange juice)

3 tablespoons real maple syrup or honey

½ cup fresh or frozen strawberries, sliced

½ cup fresh or frozen blueberries

½ cup fresh or frozen raspberries

Dash of ground nutmeg

Dash of ground cinnamon

Polenta:

2 cups filtered water, divided

2 cups nondairy milk (like soy, almond or hemp)

1 tablespoon honey

1 cup cornmeal

½ teaspoon salt

For Compote: Melt the coconut oil in a medium saucepan over medium heat. Add the juice and maple syrup and stir. Add the berries, nutmeg and cinnamon; bring to a boil. Reduce heat; simmer for five minutes. Cover and keep warm.

For Polenta: Bring the nondairy milk and 1 cup of the water to a boil in a medium saucepan. Stir in the honey. In a separate bowl combine the remaining one cup water, cornmeal and salt. Slowly pour the cornmeal mixture into the boiling liquid, stirring occasionally. If polenta mixture seems to be sticking, stir more often. Lower heat and continue to cook for three minutes, stirring frequently, scraping any polenta mixture from sides of pot. Cover and continue cooking for five to ten minutes until polenta thickens. Scoop into serving bowls and top with fruit compote.

Curried-Tofu Breakfast Burrito

fatigue fighting and adrenal support | immune boosting |
mood balancing | vegan | vegetarian

We love curry and figure we might as well have it for breakfast, too. This is a flavorful, filling breakfast that will give you plenty of energy to start your day. It's also easy to take with you on the go: Just wrap it in some aluminum foil to keep warm if you're in a hurry, and munch during your morning commute.

Yield: makes 4 burritos

1 block firm tofu (14 ounces)

2 tablespoons avocado oil

1 small onion, diced

½ orange pepper, diced

2 cloves garlic, finely chopped

1 teaspoon ground cumin

4 teaspoons curry powder

¼ teaspoon turmeric

1 tablespoon tamari

2 tablespoons fresh parsley, chopped

2 cups baby spinach, packed

4 sprouted whole-grain tortilla wraps

4 teaspoons nutritional yeast flakes

Cut the tofu into ½-inch blocks. Sauté the onion and pepper in oil on medium heat for five minutes or until soft. Add the garlic and sauté for one minute. Add the tofu, cumin, curry, turmeric and tamari and cook for ten minutes, stirring often. Add the parsley and spinach. Cover and cook for three minutes, stirring occasionally. Remove from heat and scoop into the tortillas. Sprinkle one teaspoon of nutritional yeast over top of tofu mixture and roll up in the tortilla.

Creamy Raspberry-Walnut Oatmeal

*brain boosting | comfort food | constipation kicking | fatigue fighting and adrenal support |
mouth sore friendly | nausea nixing | vegan | vegetarian*

Steel-cut oats are whole oat groats, cut into pieces traditionally by a steel blade (hence "steel cut"). Because they are a complex carbohydrate, they will provide lasting energy and likely sustain you for several hours. Adding the walnuts provides your body with the healthy omega-3 fatty acids and a good source of protein.

Yield: makes 3 cups

2¼ cups water

1 cup steel-cut oats

½ cup Sunny Hemp Mylk (page 316) or Almond Mylk (page 318), or store-bought

¼ cup raspberries

2 tablespoons walnut halves or pieces

Brown-rice syrup or real maple syrup to taste (optional)

Add the water to a pot and bring to a boil. Add the oats, turn heat to low and cover, stirring periodically until water is absorbed (thirty minutes). Stir in the hemp or almond milk and continue to cook, stirring, until milk is absorbed (about ten minutes). Scoop the oatmeal into a bowl and top with the raspberries, walnuts and maple syrup or brown rice syrup.

Annette's Tasty Tip: Try making up a large batch of oatmeal when you have more time and store in the refrigerator to reheat and eat for a few days. This saves time and creates a quick, healthy breakfast you can have on hand.

Banana-Pecan Pancakes with Chocolate-Coconut Drizzle

brain boosting | comfort food | fatigue fighting and adrenal support | mouth sore friendly | vegetarian

While making pancakes on a busy weekday may not work well, spending a lazy weekend morning cooking and enjoying this delicious breakfast is well worth it. Using whole-grain flour, such as spelt flour, make these less processed and more nutritious, so you will feel sustained longer. The chocolate-coconut drizzle is made from coconut oil and raw cacao powder. The coconut oil contains medium-chain fatty acids, which are known to improve metabolism and thyroid function, promote weight loss and boost energy.

Yield: makes fifteen 3-inch pancakes

1½ cups spelt flour

2 teaspoons baking powder

1 teaspoon ground cinnamon

½ teaspoon salt

1 cup warm water

¼ cup real maple syrup

1 egg

2 tablespoons unrefined coconut oil, melted

1 medium banana, finely diced

⅓ cup pecans, finely chopped

Fresh berries (optional)

Combine the flour, baking powder, cinnamon and salt in a large bowl. Mix the water, maple syrup, egg and oil together in a small bowl. Make a well in the center of the dry ingredients, and pour in the wet. Stir until blended without overstirring; mixture will be lumpy. Fold in the pecans and banana.

Heat a griddle over medium-high heat. Drop the batter onto the griddle by large spoonfuls, and cook until bubbles form and the edges are nearly dry. Flip and cook until browned on the other side. Repeat with the remaining batter. Serve topped with the chocolate-coconut drizzle and fresh berries, if desired.

Chocolate-Coconut Drizzle

½ cup real maple syrup
2 tablespoons unrefined coconut oil, melted
1 tablespoon raw cacao powder

Whisk together the maple syrup and melted coconut oil. Then whisk in the raw cacao powder. Drizzle over pancakes.

Annette's Tasty Tip: To save time, the dry ingredients in this recipe can be mixed in advance and stored in the fridge.

Nutty Cranberry-Coconut Granola

brain boosting | constipation kicking | fatigue fighting and adrenal support | immune boosting | vegan | vegetarian

This is a tasty and satisfying granola recipe that can be eaten as a snack or for breakfast. Enjoy the scrumptious aroma emerging from your kitchen as the granola toasts in your oven. Keep in mind that oats do not contain gluten, but are often processed in facilities that also process gluten-containing grains. If you are strictly avoiding gluten, look for packaging that says "gluten-free" so you know it hasn't been contaminated by other grains.

Yield: makes 4½ cups

¼ cup unrefined coconut oil, melted

2 cups rolled oats

½ cup slivered almonds

½ cup halved raw pecans

¼ cup raw pumpkin seeds

½ cup dried coconut, shredded and unsweetened

¼ cup real maple syrup

½ cup dried cranberries

Preheat the oven to 350°F.

Combine all ingredients except the cranberries in a bowl and stir.

Spread a thin layer on a cookie sheet and bake for fifteen to twenty minutes until light golden brown. Be sure to stir mixture two to three times during baking to avoid burning on edges. Stir in the cranberries once removed from the oven.

Kendall's Tasty Tip: Serve granola in a large bowl swimming in our Almond Mylk (page 318) or incorporate into a parfait of nondairy yogurt and fresh fruit. I often like to double the recipe and store it in an airtight container once it's cooled. It lasts for several weeks that way and also makes an easy grab-and-go snack.

Amaranth Porridge
with Raisins and Mango Swirl

constipation kicking | fatigue fighting and adrenal support |
immune boosting | vegan | vegetarian

Amaranth is a tiny grain that cooks quickly and has a nice nutty flavor. Making it into a delicious hot porridge can be incredibly satisfying and comforting when you're feeling ravenous after a chemo session or need some good morning sustenance during recovery from surgery. The amaranth in this recipe can be substituted with almost any grain, so if you don't have it on hand, try brown rice, quinoa or rolled oats. If you have mouth sores from chemotherapy, try this breakfast dish without the mango swirl.

Yield: makes 3 cups

1 cup amaranth

¼ cup raisins

1 teaspoon ground cinnamon

¼ cup Sunny Hemp Mylk (page 316) or store-bought

Real maple syrup

⅓ cup water

Flesh from 1 mango, peeled and chopped

Cook the amaranth according to the grains cooking chart on page 244 (about twenty minutes). In the last few minutes, stir in the raisins, cinnamon and hemp milk. Cook for remaining three to five minutes until the water and hemp milk is mostly absorbed, and top with maple syrup or mango swirl, as desired.

Optional Mango Swirl: Add the ⅓ cup water and mango in a small saucepan and bring to a boil. Reduce to low heat to simmer for ten minutes. Remove from heat and blend with an immersion blender until smooth, about thirty seconds. Spoon on top of the cooked amaranth and swirl into the cereal with a spoon.

Banana Veggie Muffins

comfort food | *fatigue fighting and adrenal support* | *vegetarian*

We love to make a batch of these muffins to have on hand for a snack or grab-and-go breakfast. They are filled with good-for-you veggies, heart-healthy and protein-rich walnuts, and are made with spelt flour, which is a much better choice nutrition-wise than a typical white flour. Plus they're sweetened with a whole food—bananas—instead of refined sugar. Try having a muffin with one of our smoothies for an easy traveler's breakfast.

Yield: makes 18 muffins

2 cups spelt flour

2 teaspoons baking soda

½ teaspoon salt

1 tablespoon ground cinnamon

⅓ cup real maple syrup

1 teaspoon vanilla extract

3 ripe bananas

2 eggs

1 teaspoon rice vinegar

¼ cup unrefined coconut oil, melted

¾ cup carrots, finely shredded

¾ cup zucchini, finely shredded

¾ cup walnuts or pecans, coarsely chopped

Preheat the oven to 350°F.

In a small bowl, combine the spelt flour, baking soda, salt and cinnamon. In a food processor or blender combine the maple syrup, vanilla extract, bananas, eggs, vinegar and oil. Transfer the mixture to a large bowl. Blend the dry mixture into the wet until thoroughly combined. Fold in the carrots, zucchini and nuts. Spoon the mixture into paper-lined muffin tins. Bake for twenty-five to thirty minutes or until a toothpick inserted in the middle of a muffin comes out clean.

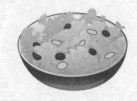

Leafy Greens

Cabbage and Cannellini Bean Sauté

brain boosting | constipation kicking | fatigue fighting and adrenal support |
immune boosting | respiratory-system support | vegan | vegetarian

Cabbage is such an easy green to add in to dishes, and it helps prevent precancerous cells from becoming malignant tumors—big bonus! This dish is simple to make, and we throw in some protein-rich cannellini beans. The combination of cumin (cancer-fighting spice) and tomato adds some fabulous flavor.

Yield: makes 7 cups

1 cup cooked cannellini beans (see chart on page 258) or canned, drained and rinsed

1½ tablespoons olive oil

2 medium yellow onions, sliced in half-moons

3 garlic cloves, finely chopped

1½ teaspoons sea salt

1 red bell pepper, thinly sliced

1 small head green cabbage, thinly sliced

2 medium tomatoes, chopped

2½ teaspoons dried oregano

4 teaspoons ground cumin

Heat the oil in a large skillet or wok over medium-low heat. Add the onion, garlic and salt and sauté until soft, about eight minutes. Add the remaining vegetables, beans and spices and cook over medium-high heat, covered, for ten more minutes or until cabbage is soft, stirring occasionally. Add salt and freshly ground black pepper to taste.

Annette's Tasty Tip: You can use this sauté as the basis for a meal. Just add some brown rice, quinoa or whole-grain pasta. You can also substitute another type of bean, tofu or tempeh for the cannellini beans.

Dandelion Greens
with Warm Tahini Dressing

blood boosting | brain boosting | detoxifying | fatigue fighting and adrenal support | immune boosting | mood balancing | respiratory-system support | vegan | vegetarian

This recipe is a super-easy side dish. The leafy green vegetable used in this recipe is dandelion greens, but any green can be substituted if dandelion isn't available. The bitter flavor of the dandelion greens is one of the flavors we should include in our diet on a regular basis (and including some bitter greens may help those of us with a coffee—a bitter beverage—addiction). The dressing contains tahini, a paste made from sesame seeds. Sesame seeds are a good source of protein and calcium. The dressing can sit covered in the refrigerator for three to four days for repeated use.

Yield: makes 2 to 3 cups (depending on size of dandelion greens)

1 bunch of dandelion greens with stems, cut into bite-size pieces 1 tablespoon olive oil 2 to 4 garlic cloves, minced	Add greens to a pan with about one inch of water. Cook for three minutes over medium-high heat. Drain water (and save for use as a stock or tea) and remove greens from pan, placing in a colander or bowl. Heat the oil in the pan and add the garlic. Cook for one minute on medium-low heat, or until garlic just begins to turn a light golden brown. Add the greens and stir in the dressing (see recipe below). Sauté for two minutes over low heat until heated through, and serve.

Tahini Dressing

⅓ cup sesame tahini

3 tablespoons tamari

1 tablespoon lemon juice

½ bunch fresh parsley

Put the tahini, tamari, lemon juice and parsley in a food processor or blender. Blend and add ¾ cup of water slowly to achieve desired consistency. Add more water, if desired.

Kendall's Tasty Tip: This is a staple recipe in our house. It has amazing flavor and you can even pour the dressing over your grains and other veggies.

Gingered Mustard Greens

blood boosting | detoxifying | hormone balancing | immune boosting | mood balancing |
nausea nixing | respiratory-system support | vegan | vegetarian

Mustard greens are light and airy and provide an uplifting energy. These greens cook down quite a bit, so don't worry that this recipe will make too much. This dish includes warming ginger and a splash of ume plum vinegar. You can find the vinegar in your grocery store near the shoyu (soy sauce) in the Asian section or order it online. We love the Eden brand.

Yield: makes about 3 cups

1 inch gingerroot, grated

2 garlic cloves, roughly chopped

1 tablespoon sesame oil

2 bunches mustard greens, chopped into bite-size pieces

½ tablespoon ume plum vinegar

Sauté the ginger root and garlic in the sesame oil in a skillet over medium-low heat, stirring, for two minutes. Add the greens and a splash of water, place the lid on the skillet and increase the heat to medium high, cooking for about three minutes, or until the greens just wilt. Drain any excess liquid and toss with the vinegar.

Annette's Tasty Tip: For grating ginger I love to use my Microplane grater. Just rinse the ginger, don't worry about peeling, and grate away! If you need to make ginger "juice" for a dish, just take the grated ginger in your hand and give it a squeeze, *et voilà:* ginger juice!

Cool Collard Green Slaw

blood boosting | constipation kicking | detoxifying | immune boosting | mood balancing | raw | respiratory-system support | vegan | vegetarian

Collard greens have a large fan-shaped leaf and a mild flavor. They make an excellent addition to soups and stews, and can be used raw, as in this recipe. They usually live in the produce section near the kale and Swiss chard. Sometimes you can find collards and other leafy greens bagged in the salad-greens section or even precut in the frozen section. Go ahead, introduce yourself and get chummy with this Food Friend! Also keep in mind that the dressing in this recipe is technically not raw.

Yield: makes about 8 cups

Salad:

1 bunch collard greens
(about 8 leaves),
thick stems removed, thinly sliced

1 large red bell pepper, thinly sliced

1 medium red onion, small dice

2 carrots, grated (about 1½ cups)

Dressing:

⅓ cup apple cider or rice vinegar

¼ cup brown-rice syrup

¼ cup avocado oil

¼ teaspoon mustard powder
(or 1 teaspoon prepared mustard)

¼ teaspoon salt

Dash of freshly ground black pepper

Combine all of the salad ingredients in a large bowl. Whisk together the dressing ingredients in a small saucepan and warm over medium heat until the brown-rice syrup dissolves. Pour the warm dressing over the collards and adjust seasonings with salt and pepper. Chill for one hour before serving.

Annette's Tasty Tip: I can just eat and eat this slaw! Talk about a simple and delish way to gobble up your greens. For an easy way to slice the collards, cut out the stem, roll several leaves up tightly into a roll (cigar shape) and then slice into thin quarter-inch strips.

Cashew Kale

blood boosting | brain boosting | constipation kicking | detoxifying |
fatigue fighting and adrenal support | hormone balancing | immune boosting |
respiratory-system support | vegan | vegetarian

Cashews give this quick-and-easy greens dish a sweet and nutty flavor and ups the protein, mineral and antioxidant content! These nuts are a particularly great source of magnesium, important for healthy bones and for muscle relaxation. You can easily substitute collards, Swiss chard or your favorite green for the kale in this recipe.

Yield: makes 2½ cups

2 tablespoons olive oil

1 large carrot, thinly sliced into rounds (about ½ cup)

2 bunches kale, thick stems removed, thinly sliced (about 8 cups)

1 garlic clove, minced

2 to 3 tablespoons tamari

½ cup raw cashews

¼ cup raisins

Heat the olive oil in a pan over medium heat and sauté the carrot for five minutes. Add the kale, garlic, tamari, cashews and raisins and sauté a few minutes until cashews begin to soften.

Annette's Tasty Tip: Double this recipe and serve on the side at breakfast to start your day with those important cancer-kicking greens!

Arugula Salad
with Raspberry Vinaigrette

blood boosting | constipation kicking | detoxifying | fatigue fighting and adrenal support | immune boosting | raw | respiratory-system support | vegan | vegetarian

Arugula is a leafy green that packs a peppery punch. Hazelnuts are a tasty source of Vitamin E and minerals like calcium, magnesium and manganese—important for metabolizing food for energy—and contain healthy fats and some protein. This salad pairs nicely with any of the soups. We especially like it alongside the Kale Pesto Linguini With Tomatoes (page 248).

Yield: makes 5 cups

Salad:

4 cups arugula

3 tablespoons pan-toasted hazelnuts, coarsely chopped

1 avocado, pit removed, sliced

1 cucumber, sliced

Dressing:

½ cup fresh or frozen (and thawed) red raspberries

4 tablespoons extra-virgin olive oil

1 tablespoon red onion, finely minced

⅛ teaspoon sea salt

2 tablespoons balsamic or rice vinegar

Rinse the arugula well and spin dry in a salad spinner. Toast the hazelnuts in a pan over low heat, stirring often until fragrant, about five minutes.

For the dressing, mash the raspberries with a fork in a small bowl. Add the olive oil, red onion, sea salt and balsamic vinegar and whisk together with raspberries. Place the greens, avocado and cucumber in a large bowl and toss with the dressing and hazelnuts.

Kendall's Tasty Tip: Mix it up and include other bitter greens in this salad. Try watercress, radicchio and endive, too!

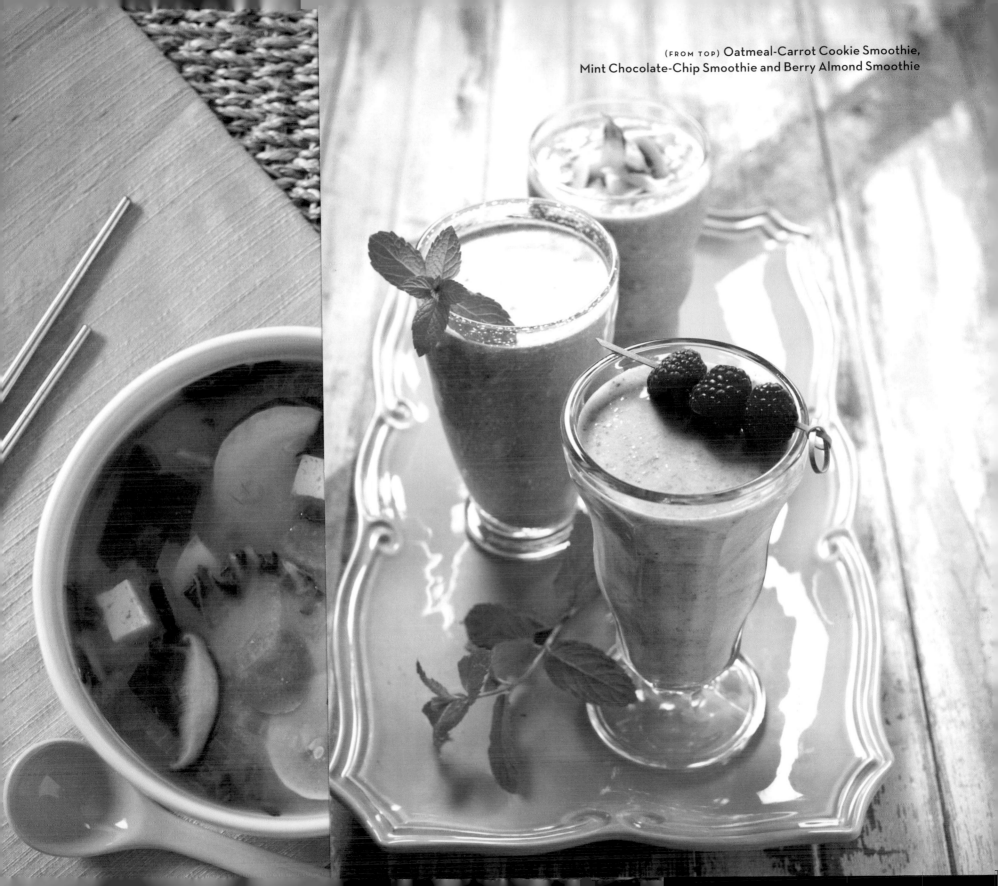

(FROM TOP) Oatmeal-Carrot Cookie Smoothie,
Mint Chocolate-Chip Smoothie and Berry Almond Smoothie

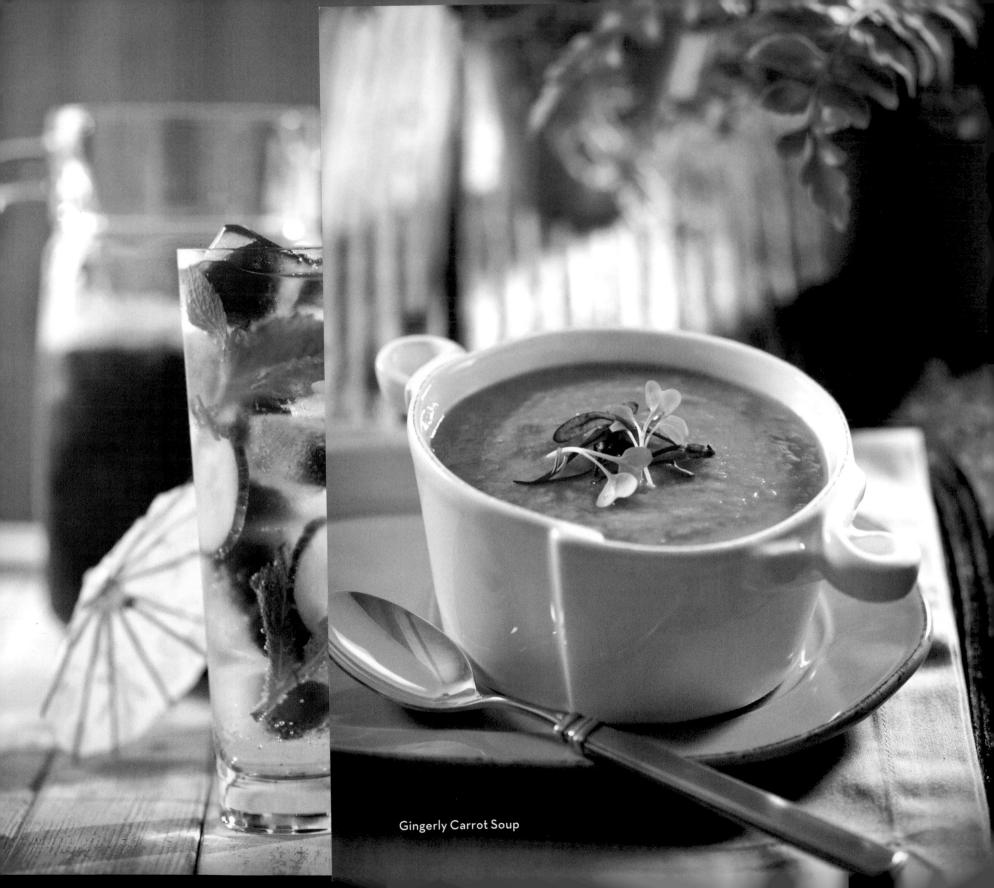

Gingerly Carrot Soup

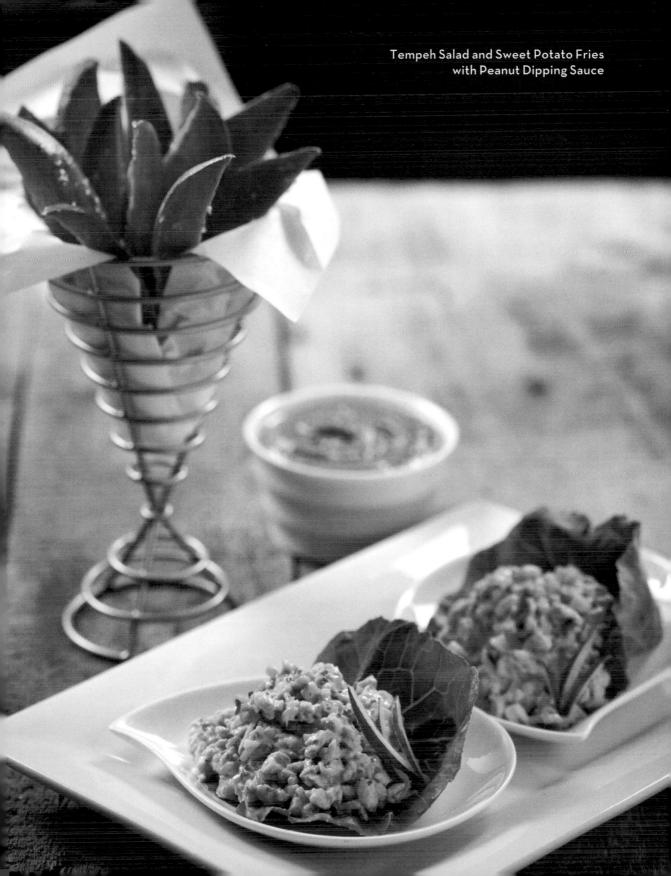

Tempeh Salad and Sweet Potato Fries
with Peanut Dipping Sauce

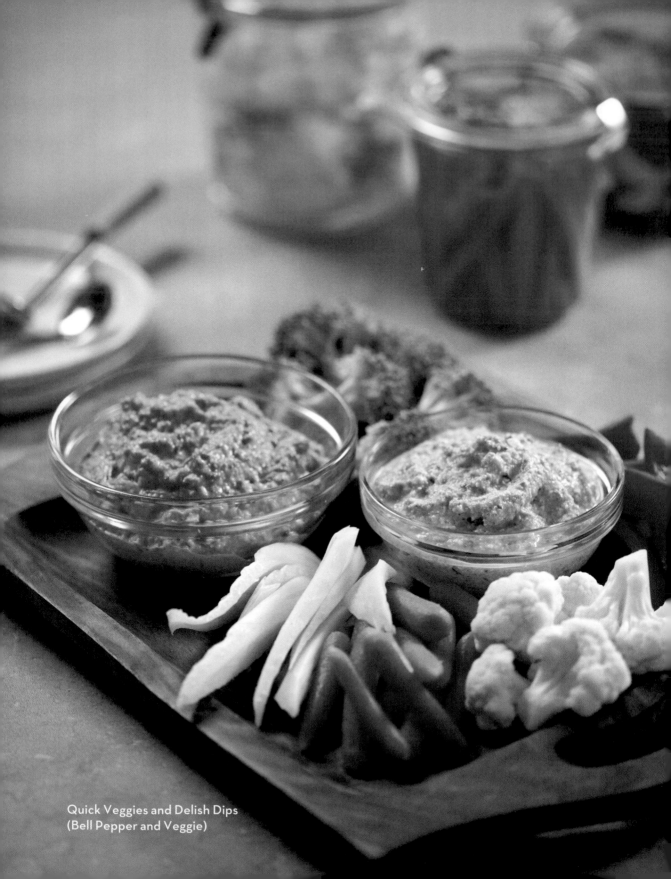

Quick Veggies and Delish Dips
(Bell Pepper and Veggie)

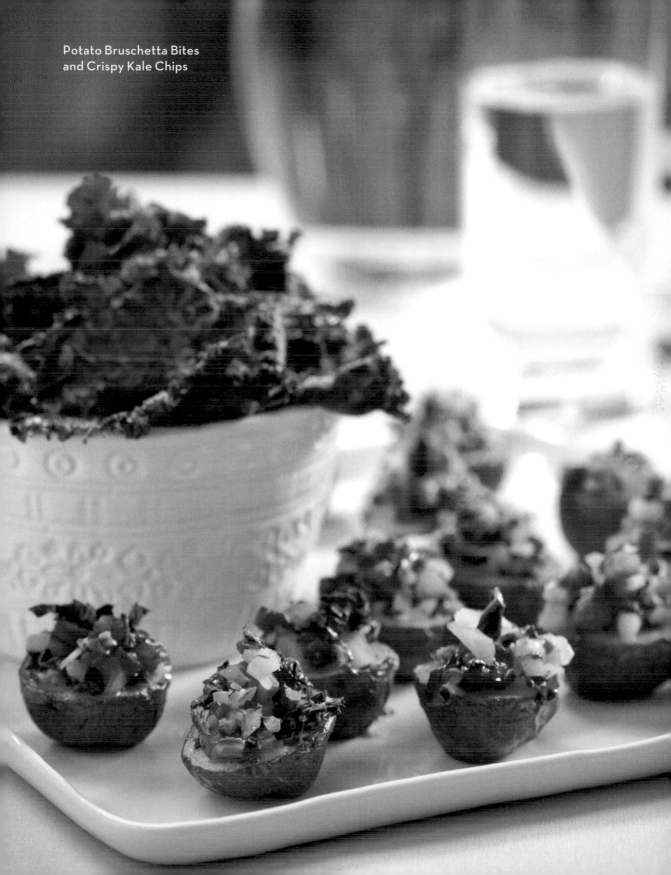

Potato Bruschetta Bites
and Crispy Kale Chips

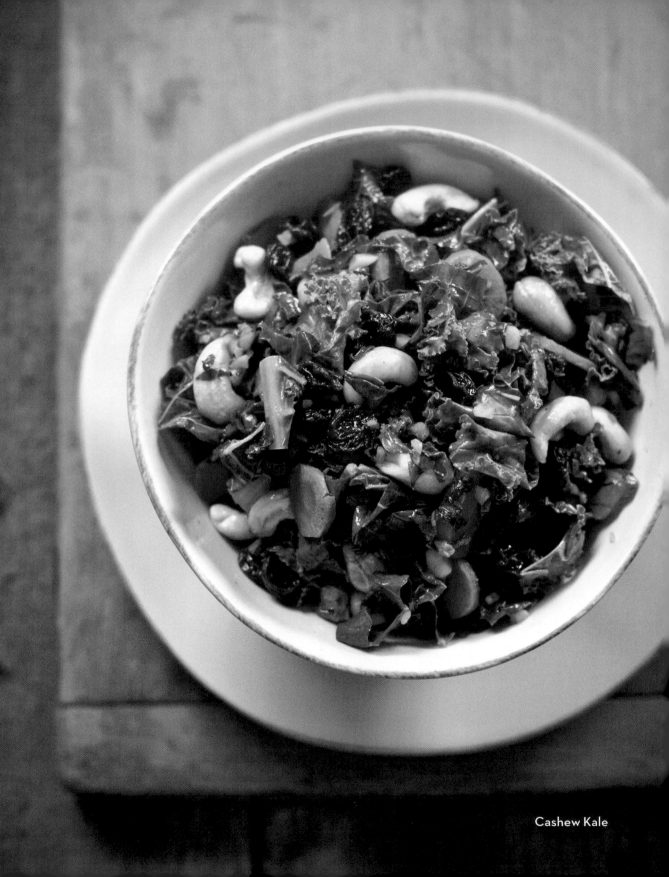

Cashew Kale

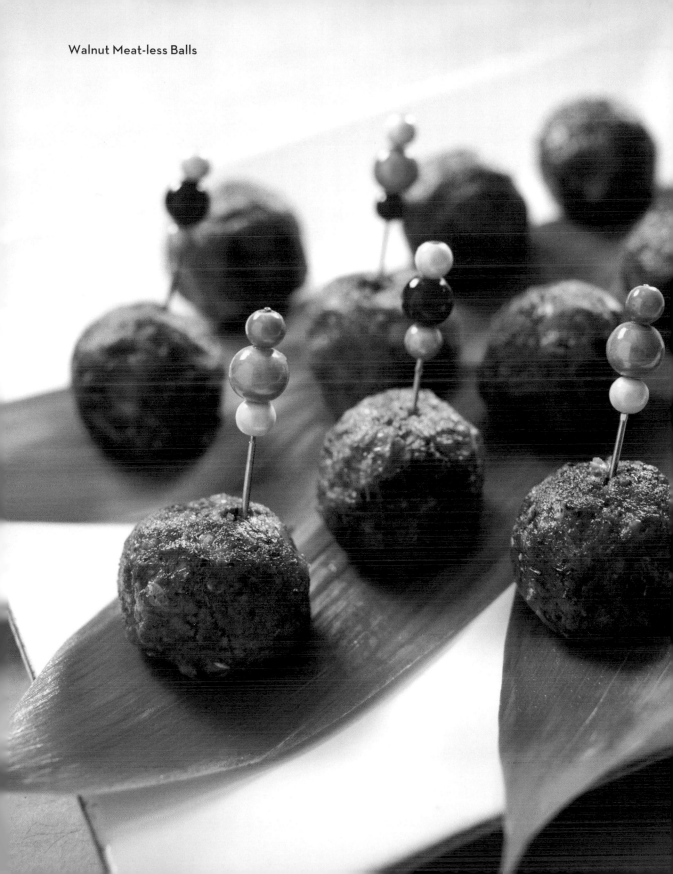

Walnut Meat-less Balls

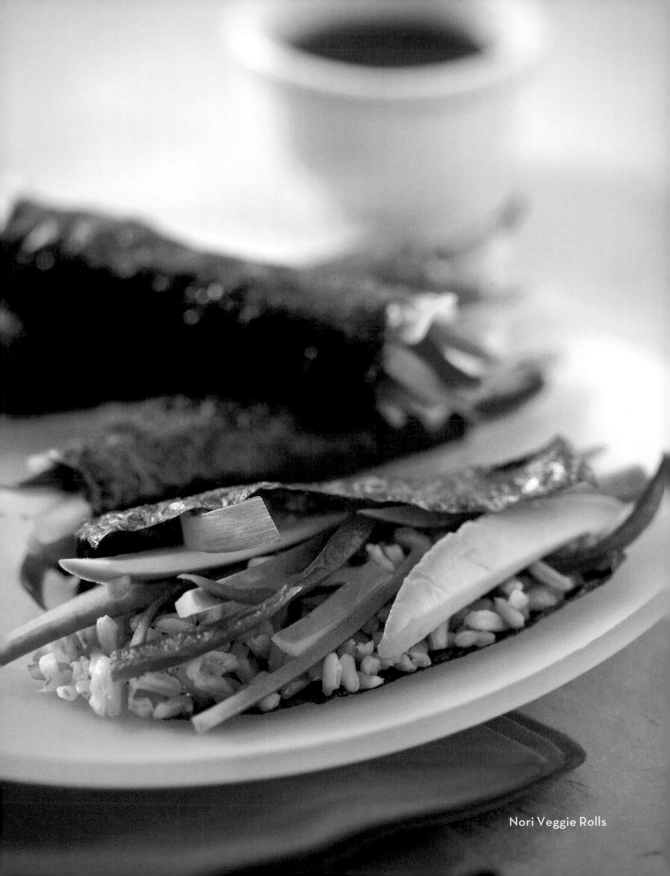

Nori Veggie Rolls

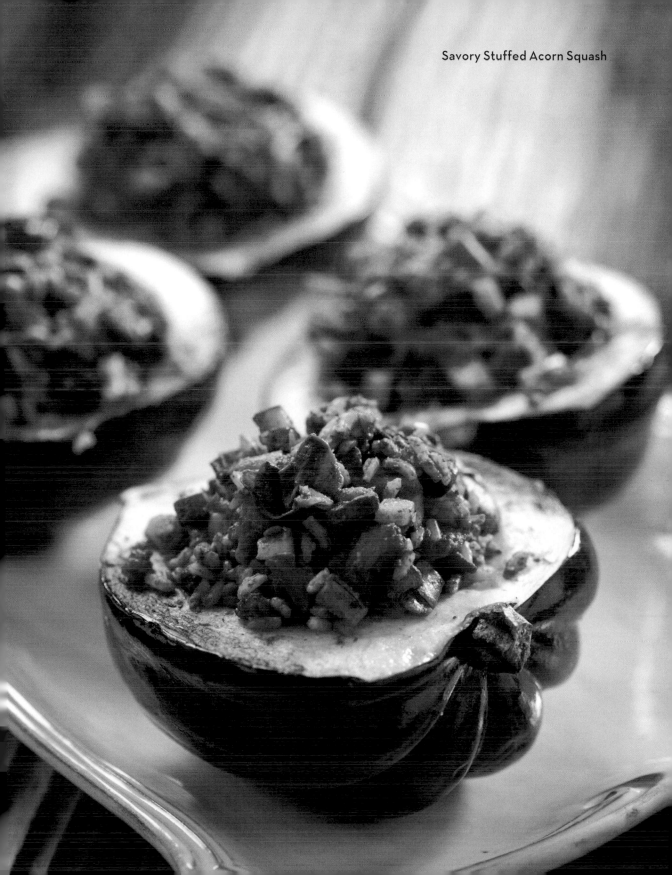

Savory Stuffed Acorn Squash

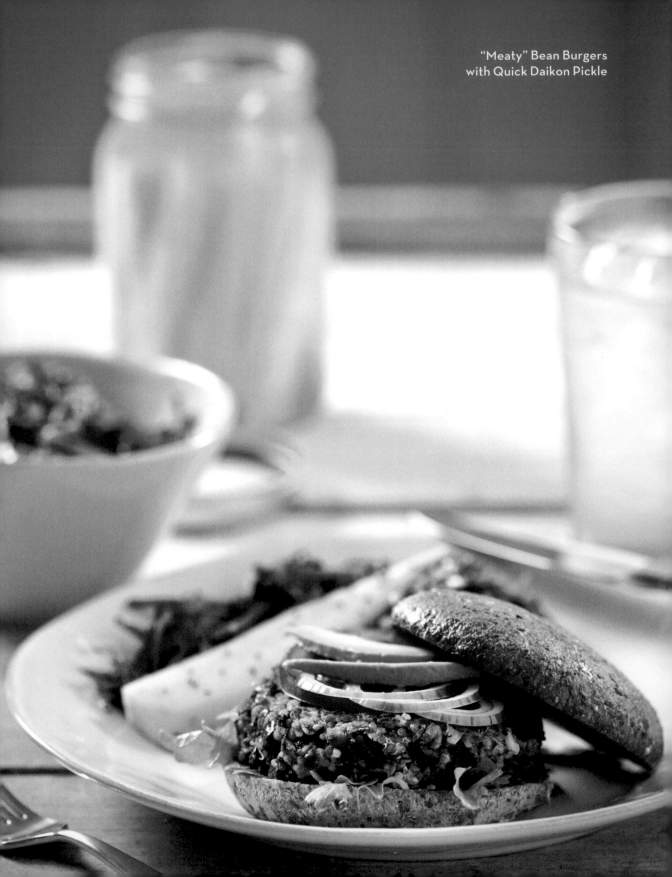

"Meaty" Bean Burgers
with Quick Daikon Pickle

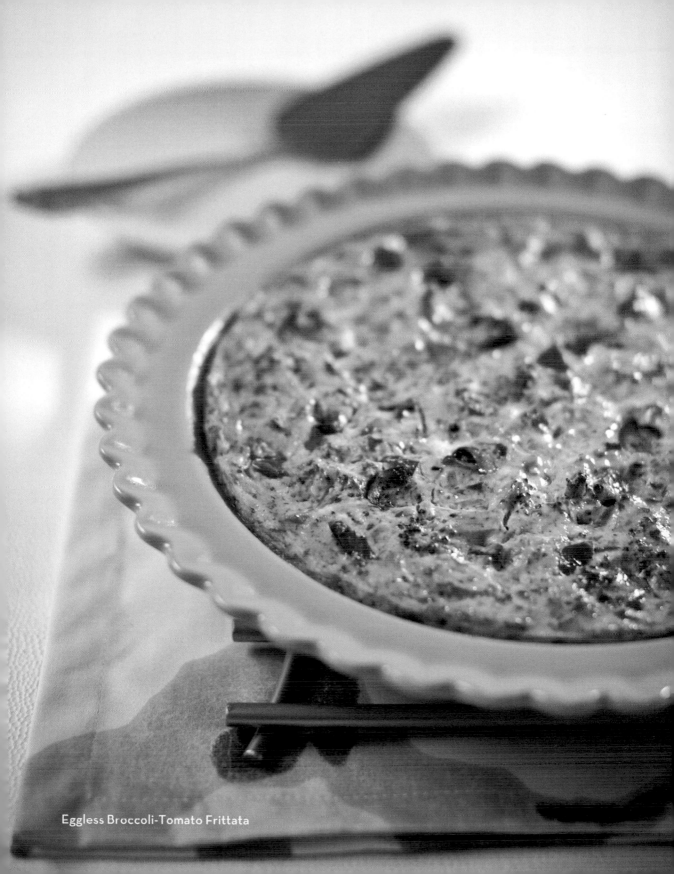

Eggless Broccoli-Tomato Frittata

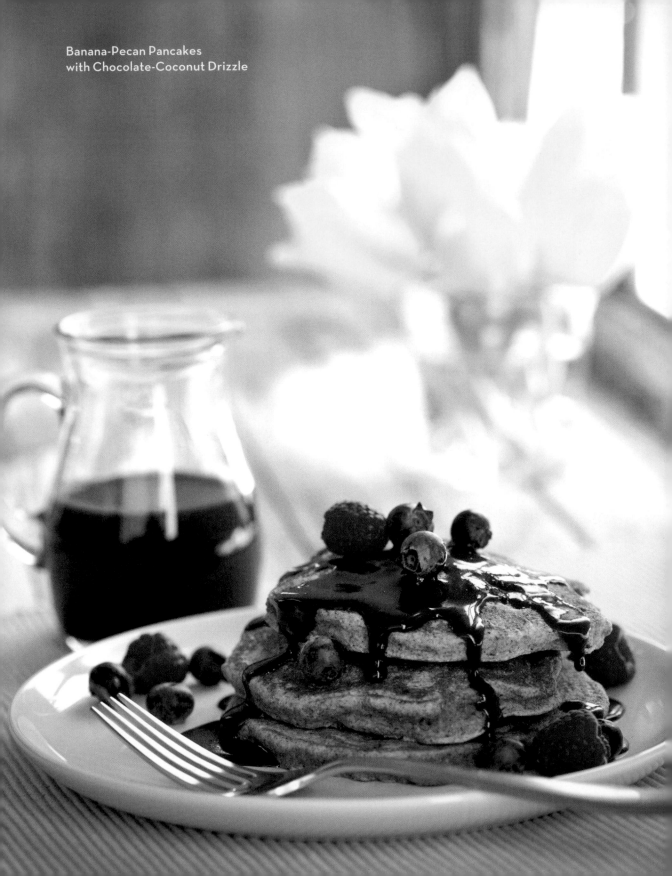

Banana-Pecan Pancakes
with Chocolate-Coconut Drizzle

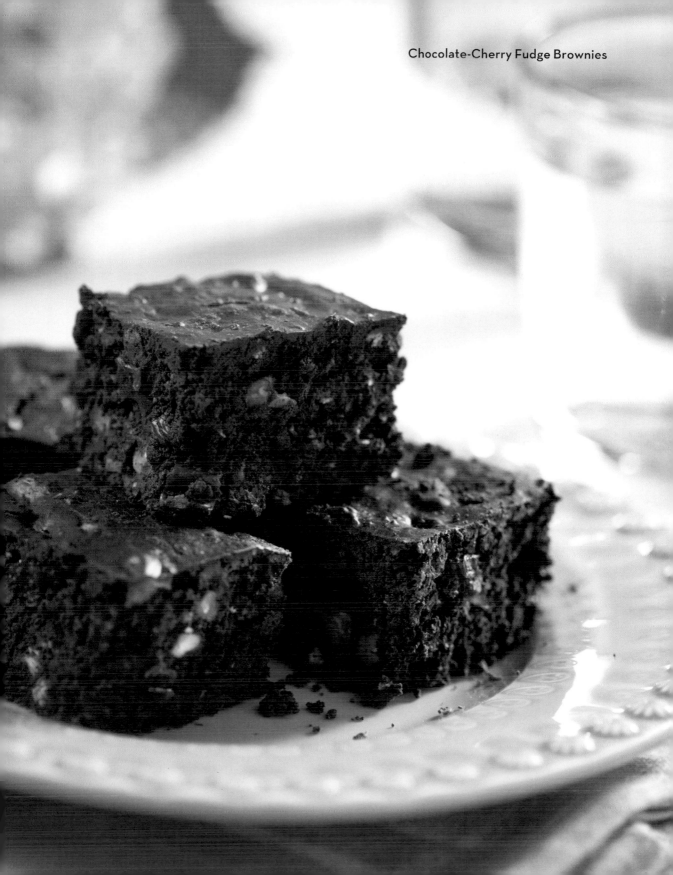

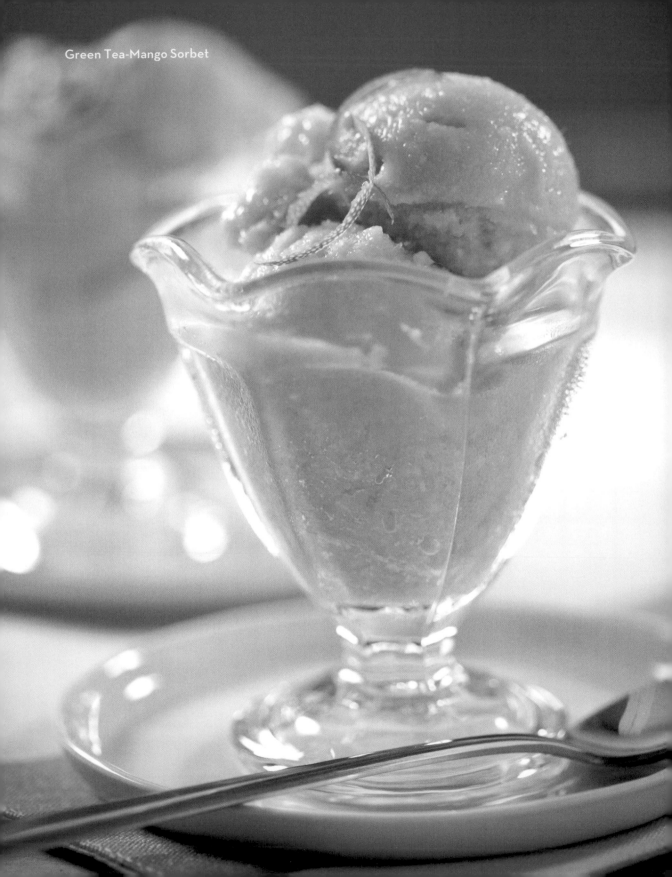

Green Tea-Mango Sorbet

Good Luck Greens

blood boosting | constipation kicking | fatigue fighting and adrenal support | immune boosting
| hormone balancing | mood balancing | respiratory-system support | vegan | vegetarian

This is a dish traditionally eaten in the southern United States on New Year's Eve or Day to bring good luck for the coming year. We've created a version that keeps the collard greens and ditches the ham bone but still leaves you with a deep, satisfying taste. And if good fortune comes your way, that would just be the icing on the cake! We love to serve this over red quinoa, a more flavorful cousin to the regular white quinoa.

Yield: makes 7 cups

1 tablespoon avocado oil

1 large onion, thinly sliced

4 garlic cloves, minced

2 teaspoons sea salt, divided

2 celery stalks, diced small

½ teaspoon paprika

½ teaspoon thyme

¼ teaspoon freshly ground black pepper

2 bay leaves

3 cups cooked black-eyed peas (page 258) or canned, drained and rinsed

½ cup fresh or frozen sweet-corn kernels

2 bunches collard greens, stems removed and slivered

In a large pot or skillet, add the oil, onion and garlic and one teaspoon of the sea salt and sauté over medium-high heat, stirring, for five minutes. Add the celery, herbs and spices, remaining salt and bay leaves and sauté for another five minutes. Add the black-eyed peas and corn and stir. Then add the collard greens and ½ cup filtered water. Place the lid on the pot or skillet and cook for five minutes, or until collards wilt, stirring occasionally. Remove the bay leaves, adjust seasonings according to taste, and serve.

Annette's Tasty Tip: Find as many ways to get leafy greens onto your plate as possible. How can you feature them in your breakfast, lunch and dinner? The more, the better!

Garlic Lover's Kale

blood boosting | constipation kicking | detoxifying | fatigue fighting and adrenal support | hormone balancing | immune boosting | respiratory-system support | vegan | vegetarian

We're always on the lookout for easy and tasty ways to get more cancer-kicking greens into our diets. Here's a terrific recipe that does just that. Garlic doesn't just repel vampires, it repels cancer, too. (But you can always skip the onions and garlic if your mouth or digestion is sensitive.) Sesame seeds, like greens, are a great source of calcium. You can boost the nutrition in this dish by sprinkling kelp granules over the onions as you sauté.

Yield: makes 2 cups

1 bunch kale, washed and chopped
(firmly packed, about 8 cups)

1 tablespoon olive oil

1 small onion,
sliced in thin half-moons
(about ½ cup)

Sea salt to taste

4 garlic cloves, minced

1½ tablespoons sesame seeds,
toasted

Fill a large stock pot about a third full of water and bring to a boil. Stir the kale into the water, cover and cook one minute, or until kale is bright green. Remove the kale with a slotted spoon to drain. Save the nutrient-rich cooking water for use as a soup stock.

In a skillet or wok, heat the oil over medium heat. Add the onion and a pinch of sea salt and sauté for three minutes, or until onion begins to soften. Add the garlic, another pinch of sea salt and sauté for an additional minute, stirring constantly. Add the kale and stir to combine. Cover and cook for two minutes or until kale is hot. Sprinkle with sesame seeds and serve immediately.

Kendall's Tasty Tip: You can make your own toasted sesame seeds. Place raw seeds in a cast-iron pan over medium-low heat. Keep the seeds moving so they don't burn. When they have a light brown color, turn off the heat. Cool and store in an airtight jar for use on grains, vegetables, salads and more.

Baby Bok Choy with Shiitakes, Pumpkin Seeds and Gojis

blood boosting | *brain boosting* | *detoxifying* | *immune boosting* | *vegan* | *vegetarian*

Goji berries have been used for thousands of years by herbalists in Asia to support the immune system. They are high in carotenoids and trace minerals as well as being a vegetarian source of protein. You can simply snack on them just like you would eat raisins. This dish packs delicious taste with a quadruple cancer-kicking punch.

Yield: makes 3½ cups

4 heads baby bok choy (about 1¼ to 1½ pounds)

5 medium shiitake mushrooms, thinly sliced (stems discarded)

3 tablespoons pepitas (pumpkin seeds)

2 tablespoons goji berries

2 tablespoons tamari

¼ teaspoon hot pepper sesame oil

Rinse the baby bok choy and then coarsely chop, separating the thick stem from the leafy parts. Place the bok choy stems in a skillet and cook over medium high heat for two minutes, uncovered. (The water from rinsing the bok choy should be sufficient for this step; if not, add a small amount of water.) Stir in the mushrooms, pepitas and goji berries and cook for two minutes uncovered. Add the leafy parts of the bok choy, tamari and sesame oil and sauté for two more minutes. Serve immediately.

Refreshing Belgian Endive Salad

dehydration defending | detoxifying | immune boosting | raw | vegan | vegetarian

Annette: This is a recipe my mother-in-law, Rosi, taught me while she was caring for me during cancer treatment. It is light, mild, refreshing and easy. Not to be confused with (plain ol') endive, Belgian endive is a mild leafy green which looks like a thin cylinder of tight, light green leaves. You can switch up the fruit you use in this recipe—so, for example, if you don't want citrus, try adding a pear or even a plum. And skip the lemon juice in the dressing.

Yield: makes 6½ cups

Salad:

1 to 1¼ pounds Belgian endive (about 5½ cups)

1 large orange

1 large apple

2 teaspoons lemon juice

Dressing:

2 teaspoons lemon juice

⅛ teaspoon balsamic vinegar

1 teaspoon extra virgin olive oil

¼ teaspoon freshly ground black pepper

⅛ teaspoon sea salt

1 teaspoon brown-rice syrup

Wash the Belgian endive and slice off about one-eighth inch from the stem end. Then, with the tip of a sharp knife, cut out and remove a cone shape about half-inch deep from the stem. Then coarsely chop the endive.

Peel the orange and cut into small pieces. Cut the apple into small pieces and toss with lemon juice (to avoid browning). Whisk the dressing ingredients together and toss with the salad.

Annette's Tasty Tip: This is a great salad to make ahead and take with you. It will hold up in transport well and keeps in the fridge for a couple of days after you make it.

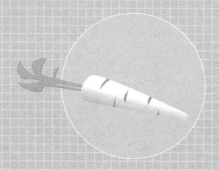

Veggies From
Land and Sea

Nori Veggie Rolls

blood boosting | brain boosting | detoxifying | fatigue fighting and adrenal support | immune boosting | mood balancing | respiratory-system support | vegan | vegetarian

We've told you how amazing sea vegetables are. Getting these kickin' vegetables into your diet will do some phenomenal things in your body. Including them in your diet a few times a week will not only be a powerful push against cancer, but also against inflammation, toxic buildup and ailments like the common cold and flu. This particular sea veggie recipe uses sheets of nori, which is a sea vegetable often used in making sushi.

Yield: makes 8 veggie rolls

½ cup brown rice, uncooked

2 sheets nori

1 small carrot

1 small cucumber

2 to 3 scallions

1 small red, orange or yellow bell pepper

1 avocado, pit removed

Tamari

Cook the brown rice according to the whole-grains cooking chart on page 244. When it is done cooking, spread the rice out on a plate to let it cool to room temperature.

While the rice is cooking, use kitchen shears or a sharp knife to cut the sheets or nori in half and then cut each half in half again, so you will have four small squares from one large sheet. Stack the squares on top of each other and set aside on a plate. Slice the carrot, cucumber, scallions, pepper and avocado into small, matchstick-size pieces.

To make the nori veggie rolls, scoop one to two tablespoons of rice onto a small nori square. Add vegetables as desired and a dash of tamari. Fold in half or roll burrito-style to eat. Leftover rice and veggies can be used for another dish, like the Fiesta Rice (page 246).

Kendall's Tasty Tip: This is a really fun meal to make with kids. My nephews love it when I make sushi rolls, and this recipe uses the exact same ingredients, but is easier to put together and you don't need a sushi mat. It's like making mini tacos with a sea veggie twist!

Savory Stuffed Acorn Squash

blood boosting | comfort food | constipation kicking | fatigue fighting and adrenal support | immune boosting | vegan | vegetarian

Kendall: I love making stuffed squash. It fills my kitchen with sweet and savory scents and fills me up without feeling bloated and tired afterward. My mother-in-law also makes her own delicious version of stuffed squash. She gave me the idea to make them up ahead of time, wrapping each half of a stuffed squash in aluminum foil, baking some immediately to enjoy now and storing the rest in the fridge for up to three days. Then you just pop them in the oven and they're ready to eat in an hour!

Acorn squash contains phytonutrients like beta-carotene, which reduces free radicals in the body.

Yield: makes 4 stuffed squash halves

½ cup brown rice, uncooked

2 acorn squash

1 tablespoon olive oil

¼ red onion, finely chopped

3 garlic cloves, finely chopped

1 small zucchini, small chop

2 medium tomatoes, roughly chopped

5 crimini mushrooms, finely chopped

2 cups baby spinach, loosely packed

1 tablespoon paprika

1 tablespoon ground cumin

¼ cup nutritional yeast

½ teaspoon sea salt

Dash of freshly ground black pepper

Cook the brown rice according to directions in whole grains cooking chart on page 244.

Preheat the oven to 400°F.

Gently scrub the skins of the squash and cut off any long stems. Slice the acorn squash in half, from end to end, and scoop out seeds and loose membranes.

To prepare the stuffing, sauté the red onion in olive oil for two minutes over medium heat or until onion begins to soften. Add the garlic and sauté for one minute until it just begins to turn a very light golden brown. Add the zucchini, tomatoes and mushrooms and cook for five minutes or until the vegetables begin to soften. Add the spinach, paprika, cumin, yeast, salt and pepper. Stir and let simmer for five minutes. Stir in the cooked rice and remove from heat.

Turn the squash cut-side up and scoop stuffing mixture into each squash half, packing it well and mounding the mixture high. Wrap each squash half in aluminum foil and place on a cookie sheet. Bake for one hour until the squash is thoroughly tender and easy to pierce with a fork.

Annette's Tasty Tip: Save those squash seeds to make a healthy snack. Place the seeds in a bowl with cool water and use your fingers to remove the squash membrane. Rinse the seeds and pat dry with a clean dish towel. Add the seeds to a bowl with a little sea salt, a dash of olive oil and any other desired seasonings, like cumin, cinnamon or garlic powder. Spread the seeds on the baking sheet. Bake the seeds at 375°F for twelve to fifteen minutes, or until they turn a light golden brown. Enjoy immediately or store in an airtight container for about one week.

Roasted Beets

blood boosting | detoxifying | immune boosting | vegan | vegetarian

In this recipe, we think you'll be pleasantly surprised with the naturally sweet, delicious flavor of roasted beets. For many of us, when we hear the word "beet" we think of the pickled beets that perhaps our grandmothers made when we were little (and we turned our noses up at them!). Fortunately, our taste buds change as we get older and flavors we may not have appreciated as kids may be quite enjoyable now. Beets can be prepared in so many delicious ways to suit our personal tastes, and it's a good thing, because they are full of vitamins A and C and magnesium, calcium and fiber. They are also awesome blood-builders, helping to detoxify and renew blood cells.

Yield: makes 2 cups

4 medium beets

½ teaspoon unrefined coconut oil, melted

⅛ teaspoon salt

Preheat oven to 350°F.

Gently scrub the beets, slice off the ends and cut into thin wedges. Lightly coat a baking sheet with coconut oil and place beets in a single layer on the cookie sheet. Sprinkle sea salt over the beets and place in the oven for forty-five to fifty minutes, or until tender. Larger pieces may need additional cooking time.

Annette's Tasty Tip: This isn't really a Tasty Tip but rather a Don't-Freak-Out Tip: If beets have not been on your plate in a long time (or ever), don't be shocked (as I was!) when your—er, umm—poo is pinkish after enjoying them. You have not suddenly developed colon cancer overnight (like I, ahem, began flipping out worrying about).

Sesame Steamed Broccoli

blood boosting | brain boosting | detoxifying | fatigue fighting and adrenal support | immune boosting | vegan | vegetarian

Broccoli has antioxidant and anti-inflammatory benefits as well as aiding in detox. Cooking it with just a little garlic, sea salt and sesame seeds is such a simple and flavorful way to enjoy this cancer-busting veggie. This can be an easy dish to go with any meal that needs some green. Try it with Marinated Tempeh Cutlets (page 259) or Simple Garlic Barley Parsley (page 247).

Yield: makes 3 cups

1 large head broccoli	Cut the broccoli into small florets, retaining part of the stem. Steam the broccoli for three minutes or until it is just beginning to soften. Heat the oil in a skillet over medium heat and sauté the garlic for one minute. Add the broccoli, sea salt and sesame seeds and sauté for two more minutes to let flavors mingle.
1 tablespoon sesame oil	
2 garlic cloves, roughly chopped	
Dash of sea salt	
2 tablespoons sesame seeds	

Fennel String-Bean Salad

blood boosting | constipation kicking | detoxifying | respiratory-system support |
vegan | vegetarian

Fennel has a mild licorice flavor as well as many health benefits including relief from constipation, indigestion and diarrhea. It is also helpful in treating respiratory disorders and anemia. This recipe also calls for radish, a cleansing, cancer-fighting veggie. Besides being high in fiber and vitamin C, studies have shown that compounds in radishes, called isothiocyanates, promote cancer-cell death.

Yield: makes 4 cups

1 pound string beans, ends trimmed

1 fennel bulb, trimmed

½ cup radishes, trimmed and sliced

2 tablespoons extra virgin olive oil

2 tablespoons lemon juice

1 garlic clove, minced

1 teaspoon salt

Dash of freshly ground black pepper

Cut the string beans into two-inch pieces and place in a steamer basket or metal colander in a pot with about one inch of water. Bring the water to a boil and steam for five minutes, until just cooked through. Cut the fennel bulb in half and thinly slice into bite-size pieces. In a small bowl, whisk together the oil, lemon juice, garlic, salt and pepper to create a dressing. Place the string beans, fennel and radishes in a large bowl and toss with the dressing.

Arame Red-Cabbage Salad

blood boosting | constipation kicking | dehydration defending | detoxifying |
fatigue fighting and adrenal support | immune boosting | mood balancing |
respiratory-system support | vegan | vegetarian

This is a power-packed salad, full of nourishing nutrients. Arame is a type of sea vegetable (or seaweed) found in most health-food stores and some grocery stores. Don't be afraid to use another type of seaweed, like wakame or hijiki, if arame isn't available. Sea vegetables are incredibly detoxifying and can be added to almost any salad, so give them a try.

Yield: makes about 8 cups

½ cup dried arame

1 head green-leaf lettuce, washed and roughly chopped

1 large carrot, shredded

½ small red cabbage, shredded (about 2 cups)

1 small daikon radish, shredded (about 2 cups)

3 scallions, chopped

Dressing:

1 garlic clove, finely chopped

1-inch piece gingerroot, grated

3 tablespoons tamari

3 tablespoons toasted sesame oil

1 tablespoon lemon juice

¼ cup toasted sesame seeds

Soak the arame in cold water for ten minutes until rehydrated. Drain and rinse. Add the arame, lettuce, carrot, cabbage, daikon radish and scallions to a large bowl. In a small bowl, combine the garlic, ginger, tamari, sesame oil and lemon juice and mix well. Pour the dressing over the salad and toss until coated. Sprinkle sesame seeds on top.

Kendall's Tasty Tip: The sesame seeds in this recipe can be toasted or raw. If you can only find raw seeds, just dry sauté them in a pan (no oil or water) on medium heat for about five to seven minutes or until light golden brown. Be sure to stir occasionally to avoid burning.

Burdock and Carrot Sauté

blood boosting | detoxifying | immune boosting | vegan | vegetarian

This dish is so delicious and strengthening! Burdock is a slender, brown-skinned root vegetable and has a firm, meaty texture which takes on the flavor of foods cooked with it. Burdock is a detoxifying and purifying food, so it helps to release toxins and promotes healthy blood production. If you can't find it at your grocery store, try an Asian market. It's worth the effort! Sautéing with carrot sweetens this dish and sesame seeds add calcium and protein.

Yield: makes 2¼ cups

1 tablespoon avocado oil

1 large burdock root, scrubbed but not peeled, sliced into coins (about 1 cup)

4 medium carrots, sliced into coins (about 2 cups)

Sea salt

2 scallions, chopped (white parts)

2 tablespoons tamari

1 teaspoon real maple syrup

1 tablespoon sesame seeds, toasted

Heat the oil in a skillet over medium heat and add the burdock and carrots and a pinch of sea salt. Sauté for five minutes, stirring constantly. Add three tablespoons of water and the scallions to the skillet, cover and simmer for ten minutes on low heat. Add the tamari and maple syrup and cook for five minutes. Remove from heat and garnish with the sesame seeds.

Oven-Roasted Asparagus and Portobello Mushrooms

brain boosting | detoxifying | immune boosting | vegan | vegetarian

For such a simple recipe, this dish packs a lot of flavor. Roasting the asparagus and porto-bello mushrooms makes them nice and juicy and they go well with a variety of other dishes. Try alongside Tahini Spinach Spelt Berries (page 249) or "Meaty" Bean Burgers (page 264). Asparagus contains folate, which helps to prevent pain and inflammation and protects against cancer. Portobello mushrooms are an excellent source of selenium, a mineral that works as an antioxidant and helps repair DNA.

Yield: makes 4 cups

1 pound asparagus	Preheat the oven to 400°F.
2 portobello mushrooms, sliced	Cut or snap dry ends off the asparagus then cut into two-inch pieces. Place the asparagus and mushrooms in a large bowl and toss with oil, salt and pepper. Place the coated asparagus and mushrooms in a shallow baking dish and roast for ten to fifteen minutes, until asparagus is tender and just starting to brown.
1 tablespoon olive oil	
1 teaspoon sea salt	
¼ teaspoon freshly ground black pepper	

Sweet Potato Fries
with Peanut Dipping Sauce

brain boosting | comfort food | fatigue fighting and adrenal support |
immune boosting | nausea nixing | vegetarian

Sweet potatoes are a naturally sweet vegetable that can help to curb sweet cravings. They are also soothing to the digestive system, which can make these a perfect food during chemotherapy when the gut can get a little out of whack. The peanut sauce adds some protein and fabulous flavor for dipping! You can replace the peanut butter with cashew or almond butter if desired.

Yield: makes 4 cups

4 medium sweet potatoes (about 2 pounds)

½ teaspoon sea salt

1 tablespoon olive oil

Preheat the oven to 450°F.

Gently scrub the sweet potato skins with a vegetable brush and slice into french-fry-shaped pieces. Toss the sweet potato fries in a bowl with the salt and olive oil until well coated. Arrange the fries in a single layer on a baking sheet and bake approximately thirty to forty minutes until edges are crisp, stirring about halfway through. Serve immediately with dipping sauce.

Peanut Dipping Sauce

1 tablespoon minced fresh ginger
½ cup peanut butter
2 tablespoons tamari
1 teaspoon honey

Add all ingredients to a blender and blend until smooth. Add water for desired consistency. Serve with the sweet potato fries.

Cheezy Turnip and Kohlrabi Sauté

immune boosting | mood balancing | vegan | vegetarian

We love the combination of kohlrabi and turnip in this recipe. Kohlrabi tastes a lot like broccoli, just milder, and turnip has a wonderful earthy and slightly bitter flavor. Both are so yummy with the nutritional yeast, which gives this dish a cheesy flavor. This recipe doesn't call for the kohlrabi greens and stems, but you can add those in, too; just wait until the last few minutes of cooking.

Yield: makes 2½ cups

2 medium turnips

2 medium kohlrabi bulbs

1 teaspoon thyme

1 tablespoon olive oil

2 garlic cloves, minced

½ teaspoon sea salt

4 tablespoons water

2 tablespoons nutritional yeast

Scrub the turnips and kohlrabi with a vegetable brush and cut into very thin bite-size slices (about 2 cups each). Grind the thyme using a mortar and pestle or spice grinder. Place the garlic in the cold oil in a skillet then place over medium heat and sauté for two minutes. Add the turnip, kohlrabi and salt. Sauté, stirring occasionally, for eight minutes or until the kohlrabi and turnip are beginning to soften. Add the nutritional yeast, water and ground thyme. Stir well to combine and cover. Cook for five to seven minutes, stirring once, until soft.

Annette's Tasty Tip: If kohlrabi bulbs are not available, you can replace them with broccoli stems. You'll need about six long stems for this recipe.

Grains

ooking grains is relatively easy, but some grains take more time than others so be sure to plan accordingly. It's often best to start cooking your grain first when preparing a meal, and while it's cooking you can prepare the rest of your food.

You may want to purchase a rice cooker, which makes cooking easier because you don't have to watch the pot to make sure it doesn't boil over. You simply measure your grain and water and press a button. Many rice cookers are made with some sort of nonstick coating in the pot, so try to find one with a ceramic or clay pot (you can read about cookware in the Poor, Better and Best Food Picks section of Chapter 5, page 112).

It's also advisable to soak your grains first, which requires some thinking ahead, but becomes very easy once it's a habit. Try to soak them in the morning, for example, if you plan to cook the grains for dinner, or start soaking the night before to cook in the morning. Not only does this reduce the cooking time, but your digestive system will also thank you: Soaking your grains in cold water and then draining and rinsing before cooking increases digestibility, and it eliminates phytic acid. Phytic acid binds to minerals and metals in the body and removes them as it leaves the body. This means that some of those nutrients you're eating to boost your health are not being absorbed and instead exit the body with the phytic acid. Not good. Try to remember to soak your whole grains in cold water for at least an hour and up to eight hours before cooking, but if you forget, don't stress about it. Kasha (roasted buckwheat) is an exception and should not be soaked.

Cooking your grains

——————— ∿∿∿∿∿∿∿∿ ———————

EACH GRAIN LISTED below has a corresponding amount of water and cooking time for one cup of the grain. You can also replace some of the water with vegetable or mineral stock. Measure the water, bring to a boil and add the rinsed (or soaked) grains. Turn the heat to low to simmer and cook for the designated cooking time. Be sure to check the grains about halfway through to determine if more water is needed. Cooking times are approximate, so some checking and experimenting will be necessary.

Want to add an extra boost of nutrients to your grains? Try cooking with a four to six-inch strip of kombu (kelp sea vegetable). While your grain is soaking up the water, it will also soak up the many nutrients in the kombu. Remove the kombu after cooking.

If the idea of cooking a batch of whole grains almost every day seems daunting, have no fear. Grains keep well in the refrigerator, so cook up a big batch to store in the fridge and use over several days. Just reheat by adding to other sautéed veggies or protein recipes, or simply toss in a pan with a few tablespoons of water or oil and cook until heated through.

Grains (1 cup)	Water	Approx. cooking time
Amaranth	2½ cups	20 to 25 minutes
Barley (hulled)	2 to 3 cups	60 to 90 minutes
Barley (pearled)	2 to 3 cups	60 minutes
Brown rice	2 cups	45 to 60 minutes
Buckwheat or kasha	2 cups	20 to 30 minutes
Bulgur (cracked wheat)	2 cups	15 to 20 minutes
Cornmeal or polenta	3 cups	20 to 25 minutes
Kamut	3 cups	90 minutes
Millet	2 cups	30 minutes
Oatmeal (rolled oats)	2 cups	20 to 30 minutes
Oats (steel cut)	4 cups	20 to 25 minutes
Oats (whole groats)	3 cups	75 to 90 minutes
Quinoa	2 cups	15 to 20 minutes
Rye berries (soaked overnight)	3 cups	45 to 60 minutes
Spelt berries (soaked overnight)	3 cups	45 to 60 minutes
Wheat berries	3 cups	60 minutes

Quinoa with Pears
and Maple Vinaigrette

constipation kicking | detoxifying | fatigue fighting and adrenal support | vegan | vegetarian

Quinoa is quite the amazing whole grain. It is packed with protein, helps detoxify the body, is high in calcium and fiber and contains B vitamins that help balance moods and support mental clarity (chemo brain, anyone?). This simple dish shows just how easy it is to include quinoa in your diet. Try it with the Gingerly Carrot Soup (page 274).

Yield: makes about 5 cups

1 cup quinoa

1 large ripe pear, stemmed and cored, diced small

2 tablespoons fresh parsley, chopped

½ cup raw slivered almonds

¼ cup extra virgin olive oil

2 tablespoons rice vinegar or apple cider vinegar

2 tablespoons real maple syrup

½ teaspoon Dijon mustard

Sea salt and freshly ground black pepper, to taste

Cook the quinoa according to instructions on whole-grains cooking chart on page 244. Once cooked, dump it into a large salad bowl.

Add the pear, parsley and almonds to the quinoa and mix well.

Whisk together the olive oil, vinegar, maple syrup and mustard. Pour the mixture over the quinoa and toss gently to coat. Season to taste with sea salt and ground pepper.

Annette's Tasty Tip: I like making this quinoa dish and storing it in the fridge for several days to have with lunch or dinner. It's perfect because then I have a delicious whole grain pre-made and ready to eat, so I can focus on prepping veggies for the rest of the meal.

Fiesta Rice

brain boosting | constipation kicking | fatigue fighting and adrenal support |
vegan | vegetarian

This recipe rolls beans, rice and veggies into a colorful, fun dish. You can mix it up by using whatever beans you have on hand and turning up the heat by adding a little cayenne. If your tomatoes are really juicy, reduce the water to just one cup.

Yield: makes 5 cups

1½ tablespoons olive oil

1 small red onion, finely diced (about 1 cup)

2 tablespoons garlic, minced

1¼ teaspoons sea salt

¾ teaspoon freshly ground black pepper

2½ teaspoons ground cumin

⅛ teaspoon cayenne pepper (optional)

1 cup brown rice, uncooked

1⅛ cups water or Vegetable Stock (page 271) or store-bought

½ green bell pepper, diced (about ⅔ cup)

½ red, yellow or orange bell pepper, diced (about ⅔ cup)

2 large tomatoes, seeded and diced (about 2 cups)

1½ cups cooked black beans (page 2578) or canned, drained and rinsed

1 avocado, pitted and sliced

Fresh cilantro, chopped

Heat the oil over medium heat in a frying pan. Add the onion and garlic and sauté, stirring constantly, for three minutes. Add the salt and spices and sauté another two minutes, also stirring. Add the rice and sauté for about five minutes, or until the rice turns a light golden brown. Add the water or stock, peppers and tomato. Bring to a boil and reduce to low heat. Stir, cover and let simmer for fifty-five minutes. Do not stir during this time. Add beans, stir and cook for additional five minutes. Serve topped with avocado slices and cilantro.

Annette's Tasty Tip: This recipe works best when you soak the uncooked rice for a few hours or overnight. Leftovers from this meal can easily be folded into a soft tortilla for lunch on the go.

Simple Garlic Parsley Barley

constipation kicking | fatigue fighting and adrenal support | vegan | vegetarian

This recipe calls for hulled barley, which is the whole grain form of pearled barley and retains a higher nutrient value than pearled barley. Pearled barley has had the outer husk and bran layers removed, which makes it cook faster, so it is commonly used in recipes. If you choose to use pearled barley in this recipe, cooking time is forty to sixty minutes. If you have the time, try the hulled barley, to get the whole food.

Yield: makes 4 cups

1 cup hulled barley, soaked overnight, rinsed and drained

1 tablespoon olive oil

3 large garlic cloves, finely chopped

1 small bunch fresh parsley, roughly chopped (about ¾ cup)

½ teaspoon sea salt

¼ teaspoon freshly ground black pepper

Cook the barley according to the whole-grains cooking chart on page 244.

In a skillet, heat the oil over medium-low heat and add the garlic and parsley. Cook for one minute and add the cooked barley, salt and pepper. Mix well before serving.

Kale Pesto Linguini with Tomatoes

*blood boosting | comfort food | detoxifying | fatigue fighting and adrenal support |
vegan | vegetarian*

Technically, linguini is not a whole grain, but you can purchase versions made from whole-grain flour and water and nothing else. And we just had to include a pesto-pasta recipe: Talk about a comfort food! Yum! This pesto is rich and creamy with kale and walnuts mixed in, so you get leafy greens and a quality protein.

Yield: makes 8 cups

1 pound gluten-free whole-grain linguini (like quinoa or brown rice)

1 cup fresh basil leaves, packed

3 large kale leaves, stems removed

1 cup raw walnuts

2 large garlic cloves, minced

⅓ cup nutritional yeast flakes

¼ teaspoon sea salt

⅓ cup plus one teaspoon olive oil

2 tablespoons lemon juice

2 medium tomatoes, diced

Cook the linguini according to package instructions.

Purée the basil, kale, walnuts, garlic, yeast and salt in a food processor. Add one-third cup of the olive oil, lemon juice and four tablespoons of water and process until the pesto is thick and mostly smooth.

Drain the linguini and leave in the colander. In the pot in which the linguini was cooked, add one teaspoon olive oil and the diced tomato and sauté for three minutes over medium-high heat. Turn heat to low, stir in the pesto and add the pasta. Toss until the pasta is evenly coated with pesto, adding additional water and olive oil if desired for consistency. Cover and let heat through on low heat for two minutes.

Tahini Spinach Spelt Berries

fatigue fighting and adrenal support | immune boosting | vegan | vegetarian

Some people who are sensitive or allergic to wheat or gluten can consume spelt without a problem. It has a much lower gluten content and is highly water-soluble, so nutrients are easily absorbed by the body, making it easy to digest. This recipe uses tahini, making it nice and creamy, and the combination of garlic, spinach, carrots and tamari soy sauce introduces some wonderful flavor. We promise: You won't want to put your fork down!

Yield: makes 3½ cups

1 cup spelt berries, soaked and rinsed

1 tablespoon sesame oil

1 red bell pepper, seeded, chopped

3 garlic cloves, finely chopped

2 tablespoons tamari

2 cups baby spinach, packed

1 large carrot, grated (about 1 cup)

3 scallions, thinly sliced

½ cup tahini

Cook the spelt berries according to the instructions for cooking whole grains on page 244.

In a skillet, sauté the pepper and garlic in the sesame oil for two minutes over medium heat, or until garlic just begins to turn a light golden brown. Stir in two-thirds cup water, the tamari, spinach, carrot, scallions and cooked spelt berries. Cover and let heat through for two to three minutes or until spinach has wilted. Stir in the tahini, remove from stove, cover, and let heat through for two minutes before serving.

Kendall's Tasty Tip: This dish is also delicious served cold, like a pasta or rice salad. Just stick it in your fridge to cool.

Roasted Buckwheat and Gravy

fatigue fighting and adrenal support | mood balancing | vegan | vegetarian

Buckwheat is the heartiest grain and is perfect in cold weather or if you need some extra energy. It's full of protein and has a slightly nutty flavor. This recipe calls for roasted buckwheat, also commonly referred to as "kasha" (and just to make it confusing, sometimes "kasha" just means porridge made from any grain, so make sure it's actually buckwheat). You can also purchase raw buckwheat groats and roast them yourself. Once cooked, buckwheat is quite soft, and with a little mashing it reminds us somewhat of mashed potatoes. Use any leftover gravy to top other grains, greens, tempeh or tofu.

Yield: makes 2½ cups buckwheat, 2½ cups gravy

1 cup roasted buckwheat (kasha)

3 tablespoons olive oil

1 small yellow onion, finely chopped

¾ cup mushrooms, chopped (any variety)

2 cups Vegetable Stock (page 271) or store-bought

1 tablespoon tamari

½ teaspoon dried sage

1 teaspoon dried thyme

½ teaspoon marjoram

Salt and freshly ground black pepper to taste

¼ cup arrowroot powder

Cook the buckwheat according to the directions on whole-grains cooking chart on page 244.

In a large skillet, add the olive oil and add onion and mushrooms. Sauté for two minutes over medium-high heat to soften slightly. Reduce heat to medium and add vegetable stock and tamari. Bring to a simmer, then reduce heat. Add sage, thyme, marjoram, salt and pepper, stirring periodically. Cover and let simmer for two minutes to let flavors mingle.

Dissolve arrowroot powder in one-quarter cup cold water and stir into gravy mixture. Cook for five minutes, stirring, until gravy thickens. Remove from heat and puree with an immersion blender if smoother consistency is desired, or leave the gravy chunky.

Stir and mash cooked buckwheat with a spoon. Serve with several spoonfuls of gravy on top.

Squashy Macaroni and Cheeze

comfort food | nausea nixing | vegan | vegetarian

In terms of cravings, pasta was at the top of our list during cancer treatment (well, come to think of it, pasta is really an anytime craving!). We wanted a way to have our mac 'n cheese without feeling like crap afterward. This dish will satisfy your carb craving and—check out the ingredient list—it's packed with nutrition.

Yield: makes 8 cups

1 medium butternut squash, peeled and cut into 2-inch pieces

1 pound brown-rice macaroni

¼ cup sunflower seeds

¼ cup walnuts

2 tablespoons fresh parsley, chopped

1 cup rice milk

¼ cup nutritional yeast flakes

1 tablespoon miso paste

1 tablespoon tahini

1 clove garlic, minced

½ tablespoon dulse sea vegetable flakes

½ teaspoon sea salt

½ teaspoon freshly ground black pepper

Preheat the oven to 350°F.

Place the squash in a steaming basket in a pot with one inch of water and bring to a boil. Steam until soft, about fifteen to twenty minutes.

While squash is steaming, cook macaroni on stovetop according to package instructions for al dente pasta.

In a blender or food processor place the sunflower seeds, walnuts and parsley, and blend until crumbly. Reserve for later use.

Add about two and a quarter cups of the steamed squash, along with the rice milk, nutritional yeast, miso, tahini, garlic, dulse and sea salt and pepper to a blender and mix until smooth. When pasta is done cooking, drain and combine with squash mixture. Mix until well coated, then pour into a baking dish.

Sprinkle sunflower seed crumble over top of macaroni and bake for thirty minutes until crumbs are lightly browned.

Curried Quinoa

constipation kicking | *fatigue fighting and adrenal support* |
immune boosting | *vegan* | *vegetarian*

One of the largest components of curry powder is turmeric. Curcumin, which gives turmeric its yellow color, is the main phytochemical found in the spice. It is anti-inflammatory and has been shown to cause cancer-cell death in the lab. Sprinkle curry powder on your grain and bean dishes to add more of this cancer-kicker to your diet. You may be able to find whole, fresh turmeric in your grocery store: It looks similar to gingerroot and can be grated into dishes or steeped with hot water to make a tea.

Yield: makes 4 cups

1 cup quinoa

1 large carrot, chopped

1 tablespoon coconut oil

1 celery stalk, chopped

⅓ cup raisins

½ cup cooked garbanzo beans
or canned, rinsed and drained

1½ to 2 teaspoons curry powder

½ teaspoon sea salt

Cook the quinoa according to the grains cooking chart on page 244.

When the quinoa is almost finished cooking, heat the oil in a large skillet over medium heat. Add the carrot and cook, stirring, for three minutes. Add the celery, raisins, garbanzo beans, curry powder and salt. Stir and sauté five minutes. Add the cooked quinoa to the skillet and mix with other ingredients.

Annette's Tasty Tip: This dish can be made without the beans and with additional vegetables, as well.

Cranberry Brown Rice Pilaf

brain boosting | comfort food | constipation kicking | fatigue fighting and adrenal support | vegan | vegetarian

If you are craving something deeply satisfying, look no further. This is Thanksgiving in a dish; it's like a mini holiday in the middle of your week. Brown rice is a delicious whole grain (once you've been enjoying it for a while, white will seem so last year) and the herbs and cranberries up the taste and the nutritional goodness of this pilaf. You can easily use extra rice left over from the day before in this recipe.

Yield: makes 4 cups

1 cup brown rice, soaked and rinsed

2 tablespoons olive oil, divided

1 onion, small dice

1 garlic clove, minced

5 medium mushrooms, thinly sliced

2 celery stalks, small dice

1 tablespoon fresh sage leaves (or 1 teaspoon of dried), minced

1 teaspoon dried thyme

½ teaspoon salt

¼ cup dried cranberries

¼ cup water

Cook the brown rice according to the grains cooking chart on page 244.

Heat half of the oil in a skillet over medium heat and sauté the onion for two minutes. Add the remaining tablespoon of oil, garlic, mushrooms, celery, sage, thyme and salt and continue cooking for five minutes. Add the rice, dried cranberries and water, stir and cook for five minutes.

Kendall's Tasty Tip: We often have this rice at Thanksgiving instead of stuffing, because it has similar flavors with the sage, thyme and celery but it's better for you. And you won't have that post-Thanksgiving bloat.

Millet Black-Bean Fritters

constipation kicking | fatigue fighting and adrenal support | vegan | vegetarian

These fritters combine two grains: corn and millet. Plus you get some tasty protein-rich black beans, making this a hearty dish. If you cook your beans with kombu, you can incorporate the softened kombu into the fritters as well. Enjoy alongside Garlic Lovers Kale (page 222) and you'll have a complete meal, perfect for any time of the day. Want to make things even easier? Make these up ahead of time and freeze for later use.

Yield: makes twelve 2-inch fritters

1 cup cooked black beans (page 258) or canned, rinsed and drained

1 carrot, grated (about ½ cup)

2 scallions, chopped

2 garlic cloves, minced

1 teaspoon paprika

¾ teaspoon dried oregano

2 teaspoons ground cumin

¾ teaspoon sea salt

1 cup millet, cooked

½ cup cornmeal

2 tablespoons avocado oil

Mash the black beans in a bowl with a potato masher or fork. Add the carrot, scallions, garlic, paprika, oregano, cumin and sea salt and mix. Add the millet, mix well, then add the cornmeal and mix well. If needed, add water, a tablespoon at a time, until ingredients stick together. Heat the oil in a large skillet over medium-high heat. Scoop out about two tablespoons of the mixture and form into about a two-inch patty, flattening between hands. Place fritter into oil and repeat until skillet is full, leaving about two inches between fritters. Flip after about five minutes or when golden brown, then repeat on the other fritter side. Drain on a paper towel.

Kendall's Tasty Tip: Try using a cast-iron skillet for this recipe to get a nice crispy crust. You can serve the fritters on their own or with a dollop of salsa or guacamole.

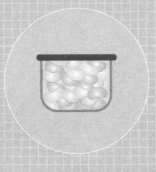

Plant Proteins

Beans

~~~~~~~~~~~~~~~~~~

Canned beans can work in a pinch, but beans cooked on your own are so much creamier and delicious. Be adventurous and try it!

Cooking beans isn't rocket science, but can take some practice. Depending on the type of bean and how old they are (tip: get yours from a store that has a rapid turnover of dried beans), cooking times and bean results may vary. If at first you end up with hard beans that just won't get soft, or beans that immediately turn to mush, don't give up. Try throwing those hard beans into a soup to cook longer, and combine those mushy beans with a grain, some crumbled tofu and spices to create a bean burger (try the "Meaty" Bean Burgers on page 264).

Store your dried beans in a cool, dry place, tightly sealed in a glass container or a jar with a bay leaf for freshness. Before cooking, sort through the beans for any small stones that might be present. Rinse the beans and, if you prefer, soak your beans anywhere from one hour to overnight and drain. Soaking beans can aid in digestibility and reduces cooking time. Place beans in a pot and add fresh water, covering to about two to three inches above the beans.

To minimize "tooting," place a one-inch piece of kombu (the sea vegetable) and a bay leaf in the pot as well. Additionally, seasonings such as cumin, garlic and fennel can be added. Then boil, uncovered, for ten minutes, scooping off any foam and floating beans that remain on the surface. Cover and reduce heat to low, cooking slowly (slower, longer cooking increases digestibility) until beans are almost tender. Then if you wish you may add some sea salt, miso, or tamari and simmer about ten minutes longer, until beans are tender but not mushy, using the following chart to reference for total cooking time. Drain.

To save time, make a double recipe then store half in the refrigerator for several days, or freeze for longer storage.

A final tip on bean digestibility: Introduce and increase bean consumption gradually, to allow the body time to adjust. Also chew, chew, chew your beans well! This will go a long way to help you and your insides love beans.

1 cup dried beans	cooking time
Adzuki	45 to 60 minutes
Anasazi	60 to 90 minutes
Black (turtle)	60 to 90 minutes
Black-eyed peas	60 minutes
Cannellini	90 to 120 minutes
Chickpeas (garbanzos)	90 to 120 minutes
Fava	60 to 90 minutes
Great Northern	60 to 90 minutes
Kidney	60 to 90 minutes
Lentils	30 to 45 minutes
Lima beans	60 to 90 minutes
Mung	45 to 60 minutes
Navy	60 to 90 minutes
Pinto	90 minutes
Split peas	60 minutes

Marinated Tempeh Cutlets

fatigue fighting and adrenal support | *immune boosting* |
hormone balancing | *vegan* | *vegetarian*

Tempeh is a traditional, fermented whole soy food, and a healthy, delicious protein choice. It can be cooked almost any way in which you'd cook meat or fish. Think of these cutlets as your piece of chicken breast and use them in a similar fashion.

Yield: makes four 2-ounce cutlets

Marinade:

¼ cup tamari

¼ cup balsamic or rice vinegar

¼ cup brown-rice syrup

¼ cup water

1-inch piece fresh ginger, thinly sliced or grated

4 cloves garlic, thinly sliced

1 package tempeh (about 8 ounces)

1 tablespoon unrefined coconut oil

Whisk together the marinade ingredients in a bowl. Cut the tempeh in half horizontally and then cut in half again vertically so that four pieces are created. Place the tempeh in a baking pan or other glass container in which the tempeh pieces fit in a single layer. Pour the marinade over the tempeh until the slices are just covered. Save any remaining marinade to use as a dipping sauce for the tempeh, grains and vegetables. Cover the tempeh, refrigerate and marinate for at least four hours.

Heat the coconut oil in a pan over medium heat. Remove the tempeh from the marinade and pan-fry until browned, about five minutes on each side. Serve with a grain and vegetable or use in a sandwich topped with sliced vegetables and avocado.

Annette's Tasty Tip: You can substitute extra-firm tofu for the tempeh in this recipe.

Hearty Navy-Bean Vegetable Stew

fatigue fighting and adrenal support | immune boosting |
mood balancing | vegan | vegetarian

This stew is full of a variety of plant foods, all offering so many benefits to your health. We often think of stews as being more of a cold-weather meal, but sometimes a nice hearty dish like this is perfect any time that you need to fill up and energize—which is often what we need during cancer treatment. Try making this stew on a lazy Sunday afternoon then enjoy it for a few days, as it stores well in the refrigerator.

Yield: makes about 9 cups

6 cups cooked navy beans (page 258)
or canned, rinsed and drained

2 tablespoons avocado oil

1 large yellow onion, diced

1 teaspoon sea salt, plus more to taste

6 button mushrooms, quartered

4 cloves garlic, finely chopped

2 teaspoons dried rosemary

1 celery rib, sliced

1 medium carrot, large dice

1 zucchini, diced

½ cup green beans

4 cups Vegetable Stock (page 271)
or store-bought

2 tablespoons dulse
sea vegetable flakes

½ cup fresh parsley, chopped

In a large pot, heat the oil over medium heat. Add the onion, sprinkle with sea salt and sauté for about five minutes. Add the mushrooms and sauté for five minutes more. Then add the garlic and rosemary and sauté for an additional minute. Finally, add the celery, carrot, zucchini and green beans and sauté for three more minutes.

Add the cooked beans and vegetable broth. Bring to a gentle simmer then allow to simmer for about ten minutes, or until the vegetables are tender but not mushy. During the last few minutes of cooking, stir in the dulse. Ladle the soup into bowls and top with chopped parsley. Add salt to taste.

Move Over Meatloaf

*blood boosting | comfort food | constipation kicking |
fatigue fighting and adrenal support | vegan | vegetarian*

Let's face it: Whether you're going through cancer treatment or not, there are times when you just want to wrap yourself up in the culinary equivalent of a warm, comforting blanket. For us, we're talking meatloaf, mac 'n cheese, mashed potatoes and, well, anything chocolate. We're pretty sure you know how to make the original less-healthy versions of these comfort foods, so we're here to offer you an upgrade. And this is one tasty substitute for traditional meatloaf!

Yield: makes 1 loaf (9 by 5 inches)

1¼ cup brown lentils

2 cups water

1 medium onion, diced

3 cloves garlic, minced

1 medium carrot, very small dice

1 small green zucchini, very small dice

1 (6-inch) strip kombu

1¼ cup quick oats

½ cup Daiya mozzarella cheese

1 cup tomato sauce, homemade or jarred

1 teaspoon dried oregano (or 1 tablespoon fresh)

1 teaspoon dried basil (or 1 tablespoon fresh)

Sea salt

Freshly ground black pepper

Olive oil

Place the lentils, water, onion, garlic, carrot, zucchini and kombu in a pot and bring to a boil. Reduce heat to low and simmer, covered, until the lentils are soft, about forty minutes. Remove from heat, and if any liquid remains drain before transferring the lentil mixture to a large bowl.

Preheat the oven to 350°F and lightly oil a 9-by-5-inch loaf pan.

Stir the lentils and all of the remaining ingredients together and combine well.

Transfer the mixture to a loaf pan, pressing firmly into the pan with the back of a spoon. Bake for forty to forty-five minutes or until the top of loaf starts to turn brown. Remove from the oven and allow to cool for about fifteen minutes before slicing and serving.

Annette's Tasty Tip: This is a family favorite in our house. My daughter asks for it all the time! It is a cinch to make and can easily be doubled. Use the leftovers in sandwiches or wraps.

Seitan Stroganoff

comfort food | fatigue fighting and adrenal support | vegan | vegetarian

Seitan is often used as a meat substitute. Made from whole-wheat flour, and often with some kombu, you can find seitan in most health-food stores in the freezer section, or in the refrigerator section with hummus and tempeh. This recipe is mouth-wateringly flavorful, and quite similar to a beef stroganoff—without the beef. You can serve this comforting dish over any grain or pasta, garnishing with a dollop of tofu sour cream. We bet this will become a family favorite!

Yield: makes about 8 cups

4 tablespoons olive oil, divided

2 medium onions, sliced

2 teaspoons sea salt, divided, plus more to taste

4 garlic cloves, minced

4 cups mushrooms, sliced (any variety)

1½ teaspoons dried thyme, minced

¾ tablespoon paprika

2 cups seitan, sliced into bite-sized pieces

¾ cup red wine (or, if in treatment, grape juice)

1½ cups cold water

2 tablespoons arrowroot powder

⅓ cup nutritional yeast

⅓ cup nondairy milk

2 teaspoons Dijon mustard

1 cup peas, fresh or frozen

Heat two tablespoons of the olive oil in a deep skillet over medium heat. Add the onions and one teaspoon of the sea salt and sauté for five minutes. Add the garlic, mushrooms, thyme, paprika and the remaining salt then sauté for five minutes or until the mushrooms and onions soften.

In a separate skillet, heat the remaining two tablespoons of olive oil over medium heat and add the seitan. Sauté for ten to fifteen minutes or until browned, flipping about halfway through. Browning is best achieved using a cast-iron skillet.

Add the wine (or grape juice) to the skillet with the mushrooms and increase the heat to high to reduce the liquid, about ten minutes. During this time, mix the cold water with the arrowroot powder in a small bowl. Then lower the heat to medium high and add the arrowroot-water mixture to the mushrooms, stirring for about five minutes or until the sauce thickens. Add the nutritional yeast and stir well to combine. Reduce the heat to low and add the nondairy milk, mustard, browned seitan and peas. Stir and cook for ten minutes to let flavors mingle. Add salt and pepper to taste.

Tempeh Salad

fatigue fighting and adrenal support | hormone balancing |
mood balancing | vegan | vegetarian

Tempeh is made from fermented soybeans and has been shown to help fight cancer. This recipe makes a delicious substitute for other deli salads like tuna, chicken or egg. Whip up a batch and keep it sealed in the refrigerator for up to three days.

Yield: makes 2⅔ cups

1 package tempeh (about 8 ounces)

1 tablespoon soy sauce or tamari

1 celery rib, diced

1 small red onion, minced (about ⅓ cup)

4 tablespoons fresh parsley, finely chopped

4 tablespoons mayonnaise or veganaise

2 teaspoons Dijon mustard

1 tablespoon rice vinegar

1 garlic clove, finely chopped

Steam the tempeh for fifteen minutes; allow to cool then crumble into tiny pieces. While steaming the tempeh, combine all remaining ingredients in a bowl. Add the crumbled tempeh to the bowl and stir well.

Kendall's Tasty Tip: I love serving this wrapped in a large collard, kale or romaine lettuce leaf, but atop tasty whole-grain bread is great too!

"Meaty" Bean Burgers
with Quick Daikon Pickle

blood boosting | brain boosting | constipation kicking | comfort food |
fatigue fighting and adrenal support | vegetarian

Looking for a powerful protein punch? These bean burgers have everything you're want-ing and more. Loaded with plant-based protein as well as fiber, vitamins and minerals (and no saturated fat or cholesterol), beans have also been shown to fight cancer. Quinoa adds additional protein, and the kale, onions and spices turn this burger into a cancer-kicking all-star! Serve alongside our Cool Collard Green Slaw (page 222).

Yield: makes eight 4-inch burgers

2 cups cooked kidney beans (page 258) or canned, rinsed and drained

2 cups cooked black beans (page 258) or canned, rinsed and drained

½ yellow onion, finely chopped

3 scallions, chopped (white parts)

2 eggs

1 cup kale, finely chopped

1 cup cooked quinoa

2 tablespoons fresh basil, chopped (or 1 tablespoon dried)

2 tablespoons fresh parsley, chopped (or 1 tablespoon dried)

2 garlic cloves, finely chopped

½ cup rolled oats

2 tablespoons ground flax seeds

1 teaspoon sea salt

¼ teaspoon freshly ground black pepper

1 to 2 tablespoons olive oil

Put the beans in a large bowl and mash well with fork. Add the onion, scallions, eggs, kale, quinoa, basil, parsley, garlic, oats, ground flax seeds, salt and pepper. Mix well by hand or in a food proces-sor to combine then shape into eight four-inch patties. Heat the oil in a large skillet over medium-high heat. Arrange patties in a single layer, working in batches, and cook about seven minutes on each side, flipping once until cooked through and golden brown on both sides.

Enjoy with or without a bun, topped with sliced avocado, red onion, lettuce and tomato.

Kendall's Tasty Tip: I usually double this recipe and freeze the extra burgers for times when I need a quick, nutritious meal. Allow the burgers to cool, then separate with wax paper and place them in a freezer bag. When you're ready to use, simply take one or more out to thaw, then warm over medium-low heat until heated through.

Quick Daikon Pickle

Yield: makes about 20 spears (1½ cups)

1 large daikon radish, cut into spear-shaped slices
1 teaspoon sea salt
⅛ cup ume plum vinegar
Freshly ground black pepper (optional)
½ teaspoon toasted sesame oil
¼ cup clear apple or white grape juice
1 tablespoon lemon juice

Scrub the daikon and cut into spears. In a bowl, combine the daikon with the salt and massage. Allow to rest for about fifteen minutes, until the daikon releases some water. Place the daikon in a colander and rinse to remove the salt. Pat dry. In a bowl, whisk together the remaining ingredients. Place the daikon spears in a glass container and cover with the vinegar mixture, adding water until spears are just covered. Place lid on the glass jar and shake. Refrigerate overnight, then serve alongside bean burgers. The pickles will keep well in the fridge for several weeks.

Mexican Bean Skillet

blood boosting | brain boosting | comfort food | constipation kicking | fatigue fighting and adrenal support | vegan | vegetarian

This is a protein- and veggie-packed dish that everybody loves—even reluctant carnivore husbands! It's easy to throw everything into one pan and let those flavors mingle. And if you're daring, throw in the optional cayenne, and adjust to your preferred level of heat!

Yield: makes 4 cups

1 tablespoon olive oil

1 medium onion, diced (about 1 cup)

1 small bell pepper (red, orange, or yellow), thinly sliced (about 1 cup)

3 garlic cloves, minced

1 teaspoon sea salt

2 tablespoons ground cumin

1 teaspoon paprika

⅛ teaspoon cayenne pepper (optional)

2 cups cooked beans (try one cup each of black and pinto)

½ cup each of veggie add-ins, for example diced zucchini and chopped spinach

1½ cups diced tomatoes

¼ cup fresh cilantro, chopped

In a skillet, sauté the onion, pepper and garlic and salt in the olive oil over medium heat for five minutes, stirring. Then add the spices and sauté another two minutes. Next add the beans, veggie add-ins and tomatoes. Simmer for fifteen minutes, then add the cilantro and simmer for an additional two minutes.

Annette's Tasty Tip: You can also serve this dish in a sprouted whole-grain wrap with lettuce, tomatoes, nutritional yeast and guacamole.

Sweet and Strong Adzuki Beans

blood boosting | constipation kicking | fatigue fighting and adrenal support |
mouth sore friendly | vegan | vegetarian

Adzuki beans are small but mighty! Low in fat but extremely strengthening, these beans pack a protein and potassium punch. They are energizing, nutrient-dense and contain plenty of fiber. Cooking adzukis with onions and sweet potato makes this dish sweet and satisfying.

Yield: makes 3⅔ cups

1 cup dried adzuki beans, rinsed

1 small sweet onion, diced (about ¾ cup)

1 medium sweet potato, scrubbed and diced (about 1½ cups)

1-inch piece of kombu

1½ teaspoons sea salt

Place all the ingredients except salt with three cups of filtered water in a heavy pot and bring to a boil. Reduce the heat to low and simmer until the beans are almost tender, about forty-five minutes. Add the sea salt and simmer for an additional fifteen minutes. Drain any remaining liquid, remove the kombu (or not) and serve.

Annette's Tasty Tip: You can personalize the flavor of this dish by adding tamari, ginger, toasted sesame seeds or a splash of vinegar. Serve over or alongside brown rice and some greens for a cancer-kicking, strengthening meal.

Tamari-Infused Tofu on Braised Bok Choy

blood boosting | fatigue fighting and adrenal support | immune boosting | vegan | vegetarian

Bok choy, also called Chinese cabbage, is a member of the cruciferous veggie family, a consummate cancer-kicking clan. Bok choy has long white stalks attached at the bottom, like celery, with green leafy tops. It is a good source of vitamins and minerals such as calcium and potassium. It can be sliced into salads, or used in a quick stir fry, as in this dish. Make sure to separate the stalks and wash them well to remove soil that often lingers on the stems.

Yield: makes 5 cups of bok choy and 8 pieces of tofu

1 package organic extra-firm tofu (10 to 16 ounces)

4 tablespoons tamari, divided

2 tablespoons of avocado oil, divided

1 package cremini mushrooms, quartered (8 ounces)

1 package maitake mushrooms, broken into bite-sized pieces (3½ ounces)

Sea salt

1½ pounds bok choy, sliced thinly, white and green parts kept separate

Toasted sesame seeds

Slice tofu horizontally into three equal slices. Cut each slice into three equal pieces. Place the tofu pieces in a glass baking dish and drizzle with two tablespoons tamari. Allow to marinate for at least twenty minutes, turning the tofu to expose all sides to the tamari. In a skillet, heat one tablespoon of the oil over medium-high heat and cook the marinated tofu until lightly browned on each side, about five minutes per side.

Heat the remaining oil in a wok or large skillet over medium-high heat. Add the mushrooms and a pinch of salt and sauté, stirring occasionally, for three minutes. Add the remaining tamari and sauté for another two minutes. Add the white part of the bok choy, stir, and sauté for five minutes. Then add the green part of the bok choy, stir, cover and braise for three minutes.

Place several spoonfuls of the bok choy and mushrooms on a plate and cover with a slice or two of tofu. Garnish with toasted sesame seeds.

Kendall's Tasty Tip: If you can't find maitakes, feel free to substitute any mushrooms you have on hand: Try button, shiitakes and portabellas.

Walnut Meat-less Balls

*brain boosting | comfort food | fatigue fighting and adrenal support |
immune boosting | vegan | vegetarian*

These meatballs are flavorful and replicate a traditional meatball quite nicely, but without the heaviness that comes from the meat. You get a nice punch of protein from the walnuts and immune-boosting benefits from the mushrooms, onions, garlic and parsley. You can throw these into a typical tomato sauce and serve over pasta (and try using brown rice or quinoa pasta), or they go deliciously with the gravy in Roasted Buckwheat and Gravy (page 250).

Yield: makes 1 dozen balls

1 tablespoon plus
¼ teaspoon olive oil

½ medium yellow onion, chopped

6 button mushrooms,
chopped (about 1 cup)

2 garlic cloves, finely chopped

1 cup walnuts

2 tablespoons tomato paste

¼ cup fresh parsley, chopped

2 tablespoons wheat germ

3 tablespoons quick oats

2 teaspoons tamari

½ teaspoon dried thyme

½ teaspoon paprika

½ teaspoon onion powder

1 tablespoon nutritional yeast

1 teaspoon freshly ground
black pepper

Preheat oven to 375°F.

In a frying pan, heat the olive oil over medium heat. Sauté the onion, mushrooms and garlic for about four minutes, or until soft. Transfer the sauteed onions, mushrooms and garlic to a food processor; add all remaining ingredients and blend until smooth. Form into small balls (about the size of a golf ball) and place on a lightly oiled cookie sheet. Bake covered for thirty minutes. Then uncover, flip meatballs and bake for an additional ten minutes uncovered. Let them cool for five to ten minutes before serving.

Kendall's Tasty Tip: These also make great party hors d'oeuvres—and when you're feeling up to it, have a little get-together just to celebrate you. Just arrange the meatless balls on a platter with some toothpicks and set them out for the guests to enjoy.

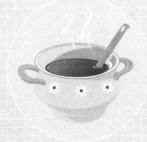

Soups and Stocks

Vegetable Stock

*dehydration defending | detoxifying | nausea nixing |
respiratory-system support | vegan | vegetarian*

Making your own vegetable broth is easy and it makes good use of raw veggie scraps. Save scraps such as tops of carrots, beets, parsnips, radishes and other root vegetables;, onion, garlic and potato peels; cabbage cores and the outer leaves; and broccoli, kale, collard and celery stems. Your broth will be full of vitamins and minerals, and will only contain the ingredients you added, and nothing artificial or processed.

Yield: makes 2 quarts

4 cups vegetable scraps

Fresh herbs or herb scraps as desired (thyme, rosemary, parsley, oregano, basil)

8 cups water

Add the vegetable scraps and the herbs to the water in a stockpot. Bring to a boil, then reduce heat to low and simmer uncovered for about forty-five minutes. Pour the stock through a colander, using a large bowl to collect the liquid. Use immediately, or pour into containers to refrigerate for up to three days or to freeze.

Annette's Tasty Tip: Pour your vegetable stock into ice cube trays to freeze. Then throw a couple into different dishes as they cook, like rice or veggie sautés.

Mineral Stock

blood boosting | dehydration defending | fatigue fighting and adrenal support | immune boosting |

Normally you won't find us cooking a recipe with an ingredient like marrow bones. Special circumstances call for special measures, however, and stressful times like surgery and chemotherapy are special. We would turn to this mineral broth for a boost when our bodies were taking a tough hit, when we were extremely fatigued and blood counts were low. It provides blood-cell and immune-system support from the marrow bones, as well as from the other powerful ingredients like astragalus, sea veggies, herbs and mushrooms. Of course, if you prefer not to use the marrow bones, simply omit them.

Yield: makes 2 quarts

Marrow bones (organic, grass fed)

Dried astragalus

Dried mushrooms such as shiitake, maitake, reishi

Kombu

Onions

Fresh herbs as desired (thyme, rosemary, parsley)

8 cups water

1 tablespoon rice vinegar

Place all ingredients in a crock pot and cook on low overnight. Pour the stock through a colander into a large bowl to collect the liquid. Allow it to cool and skim any fat off the top. Use immediately, or pour into containers to refrigerate for up to three days or freeze.

Annette's Tasty Tip: You can up the nutritional content of grain dishes, soups and stews by incorporating some of this mineral broth in place of some of the water in those dishes.

Dilly Lentil Soup

constipation kicking | dehydration defending | fatigue fighting and adrenal support | mouth sore friendly | vegan | vegetarian

This soup packs a protein punch, and with lots of fiber, it gets your digestion moving. You can choose either green (brown in color) or French (tiny and dark) lentils for this soup. Feel free to add whatever root veggies you have on hand: diced carrots, turnips, squash and potatoes go well, or toss in fresh or frozen peas or sweet corn.

Yield: makes 8 cups

1 cup lentils

3 cups of one or more root vegetables, small dice

2 bay leaves

2 garlic cloves, finely chopped

4 tablespoons dried dill

1 teaspoon ground cumin

1 teaspoon sea salt

½ teaspoon dried thyme, ground

5 cups water or Vegetable Stock (page 271) or store-bought

3 tablespoons lemon juice

Add all the ingredients except the lemon juice to a stockpot. Bring to a boil then reduce heat to low and simmer for twenty to thirty minutes, or until the lentils are tender. Stir in the lemon juice and remove the bay leaves.

Annette's Tasty Tip: Give your lentils a rinse before using, and scan for and remove any little pebbles that may have found their way into the bag.

Gingerly Carrot Soup

blood boosting | dehydration defending | nausea nixing | vegan | vegetarian

This soup can be enjoyed warm or cold, depending on the time of the year. The flavors mingle the longer they hang out together, so cook it well ahead of time if possible. Feel free to adjust the amount of ginger for a milder or stronger flavor. Cancer-fighting miso helps strengthen the good bacteria in the gut, and adds a little saltiness. Enjoy alongside the Arugula Salad With Raspberry Vinaigrette on page 224.

Yield: makes 5 cups

2 tablespoons olive oil

1 large sweet onion, chopped

1 leek, well rinsed and sliced in rings

Sea salt

2-inch piece fresh ginger, finely grated

½ teaspoon ground cinnamon

1 pound carrots, scrubbed with ends removed, and chopped

Juice of one orange

2 to 3 cups vegetable stock

1 tablespoon miso

Freshly ground black pepper

In a stockpot, heat the oil over medium heat. Add the onion, leek and a pinch of sea salt and sauté until the onion is soft, about five minutes. Add the ginger and cinnamon and sauté another 5 minutes, stirring constantly.

Add the carrots, orange juice and enough stock to cover the carrots. Bring to a boil; reduce heat then simmer, covered, until carrots are tender enough to pierce with a fork, about twenty minutes.

Turn off the heat, and purée with an immersion blender. Remove a small amount of the soup (about ½ cup) and mix it with the miso in a small bowl. Add miso mixture to the soup and warm on low heat for several minutes. Check a spoonful for seasoning, adding pepper as needed.

Annette's Tasty Tip: This is a wonderful soup to pack in a thermos on treatment days when you want to eat something soothing and easy on the stomach.

Mighty Mushroom Soup

blood boosting | brain boosting | dehydration defending | immune boosting |
mouth sore friendly | vegan | vegetarian

Mushrooms offer a terrific boost to the immune system as well as a satisfying, deep flavor. Herbs are powerful cancer-kickers: Use them to boost the nutritional value of whatever you are cooking, and to personalize your dish. Feel free to make this easy soup recipe your own, and have fun with it by changing up the types of mushrooms and herbs you use.

Yield: makes about 8 cups

3 tablespoons olive oil, divided

2 large yellow or white onions, chopped

2 cloves of garlic, roughly chopped

Sea salt

1 large carrot, chopped

2 small potatoes, diced with skins on

2 ribs celery, diced

4 cups water or vegetable stock

2 tablespoons tamari

1 pound mushrooms, cut into bite-size pieces (try button, portabella, maitake or shiitake)

1 tablespoon dried rosemary

1 teaspoon dried sage

2 tablespoons fresh parsley, chopped

Heat half the oil in a stockpot. Add the onions, garlic and a couple of pinches of salt. Cover and cook over medium heat until the onions are soft, about five minutes. Add the carrot, potatoes, celery and water or veggie stock; cover and simmer until the vegetables are tender, about fifteen minutes. Remove from heat and purée until smooth using an immersion blender. Add the tamari.

Heat the remaining half of the oil in a skillet and sauté the mushrooms with a pinch of salt and the herbs until just soft. Add the mushroom mixture to the soup.

Kendall's Tasty Tip: I loved this soup while going through treatment when I wanted something hearty and flavorful but still easy to swallow. What better way to get all that, along with great nutrition?

Curried Red-Lentil Soup

dehydration defending | fatigue fighting and adrenal support |
mouth sore friendly | vegan | vegetarian

An excellent source of protein, red lentils cook up quickly and make a terrific addition to this veggie-rich soup. Leeks belong to the same family as onions and garlic, with a mild taste. They offer numerous nutritional benefits, from vitamins C, K and A to sulfur, manganese, calcium and magnesium. Use the light-colored part of the leek and slice it down the middle, rinsing it very well under running water to remove any dirt. Curry powder contains turmeric, a star in the cancer-kicking spice world.

Yield: makes about 8 cups

2 cups red lentils

2 tablespoons olive oil

1 large onion, finely chopped

2 cloves garlic, finely chopped

Sea salt

2½ tablespoons curry powder

2 large carrots, diced

1 celery root, diced

5 cups Vegetable Stock (page 271) or store-bought

1 leek, cut into thin rings

2 tablespoons tamari

Freshly ground black pepper

1 tablespoon lemon juice

Fresh parsley, chopped for garnish

Rinse the lentils in a fine mesh strainer. Heat the olive oil in a stockpot and sauté the onion, garlic and a pinch or two of sea salt for about five minutes or until the onion is soft. Then add the curry powder and sauté for one minute until the curry is well blended. Add the carrots, celery root, lentils and vegetable stock or water. Bring to a boil and then reduce heat to simmer for ten minutes. Add the leek and simmer for ten more minutes or until the vegetables and lentils are tender. Add the tamari, sea salt, pepper and lemon juice to taste, and serve topped with fresh parsley.

Annette's Tasty Tip: Celery root, also called celeriac, can usually be found in the fresh vegetable section near the turnips and beets. It is round and knobby in shape, with a white color often shaded brown from soil. It can either be scrubbed or peeled. Celery root is a good source of fiber, vitamin B6, magnesium and manganese, and a great source of vitamin C, vitamin K, phosphorus and potassium.

Potato Leek Soup

comfort food | mouth sore friendly | nausea nixing | vegan | vegetarian

If you are craving comfort food, try this creamy, delicious soup. It satisfies the desire for starchy carbohydrates we often have during chemo (or anytime!) but adds the nutritional value found in the potato skins and in the leeks and garlic. Try this soup with Gingered Mustard Greens (page 221).

Yield: makes 8 cups

2 tablespoons olive oil

4 leeks, white portion, well rinsed and cut into thin rings

Pinch of sea salt

1 garlic clove, minced

6 medium potatoes, scrubbed and diced

1 quart Vegetable Stock (page 271) or store-bought

2 tablespoons organic butter (optional)

1 cup nondairy milk

Dash of ground nutmeg

Freshly ground white pepper

Add the olive oil to a stockpot over medium heat. Add the leeks and a pinch of salt and sauté for ten minutes, stirring occasionally. Add the garlic and sauté for an additional three to four minutes. Add the potatoes and vegetable broth, and bring to a boil over medium-high heat. Reduce the heat to low and cover. Simmer for thirty minutes until the potatoes are cooked through. Remove from the heat and use a handheld immersion blender to blend the soup until smooth. Stir in the butter (if using), nondairy milk, nutmeg and white pepper.

Kendall's Tasty Tip: To get your leafy greens, add some chopped, fresh kale to the soup during the last few minutes of cooking and before blending.

Creamy Broccoli Soup

constipation kicking | fatigue fighting and adrenal support | immune boosting |
mouth sore friendly | vegan | vegetarian

We love an easy soup, and this one takes almost no time to make, with only a few ingredients. It includes a green veggie, a whole grain and protein-boosting miso. There's no cheese or other dairy that are in many cream-based soups, so this is indeed a vegan soup that you'll love!

Yield: makes 9 cups

1 bunch broccoli (about 1 pound)

1 small cauliflower (about 1 pound)

6 cups Vegetable Stock (page 271) or store-bought

1 onion, chopped

2 garlic cloves, minced

3 tablespoons miso

1 cup cooked brown rice

2 tablespoons fresh parsley, chopped

1 teaspoon salt

¼ teaspoon ground black or white pepper

Wash the broccoli and separate stems from florets. Chop the stems and create bite-sized floret pieces. Reserve one cup of the floret pieces. Wash the cauliflower and chop. In a stockpot, bring the vegetable stock to a boil. Add the broccoli stems, unreserved florets, cauliflower, onion and garlic. Reduce heat and simmer for fifteen minutes.

Remove one cup of liquid from the pot then dissolve miso paste in this liquid, using a whisk. Return the miso mixture to the pot. Add the brown rice and parsley. Use a handheld immersion blender to purée the soup. Add the reserved broccoli florets and simmer ten more minutes.

Kendall's Tasty Tip: My husband and I both love a traditional cheese and broccoli soup, but prefer not to have the cheese and heavy cream. This is a delicious alternative that give us energy and fills us up without being too heavy. Use leftover rice from the day before to make this recipe even easier.

Marvelous Miso Soup

blood boosting | dehydration defending | detoxifying | fatigue fighting and adrenal support | immune boosting | mood balancing | mouth sore friendly | nausea nixing | vegan | vegetarian

Miso is created by mixing a blend of rice, barley or soybeans with the fungus Aspergillus oryzae and salt and allowing the mixture to ferment before grinding it into a thick paste. High in vitamins, minerals and protein, miso is easily incorporated into your cooking instead of salt and provides nutritional benefits and enhanced flavor. There are many varieties to choose from, ranging in color from light to dark and in taste from delicate to more intense. Try a combination of light and dark: For example, you can use four tablespoons of chickpea miso and two tablespoons of barley miso in this recipe. In addition to the miso, the sea and land veggies give this soup all-star cancer-kicking status.

Yield: makes 8 cups

5-inch strip kombu

1 small onion, sliced in half-moons (about 1 cup)

5 shiitake mushrooms, finely sliced (about 1 cup)

6 cups water

1 medium carrot, thinly sliced (about ⅓ cup)

1 baby bok choy, chopped (about 1 cup)

1 small yellow squash, halved then sliced in half-moons (about 1 cup)

1 teaspoon dried wakame, rehydrated in water then finely diced

1 cup cubed tofu (optional)

6 tablespoons miso

Place the kombu, onion, mushrooms and water in a stockpot. Bring to a boil and reduce heat to low, simmering for twenty minutes. Remove the kombu and add the vegetables, wakame and tofu. Simmer for ten minutes. Turn heat off. Remove about a half cup of the broth and add to the miso in a bowl, mixing with a whisk or pestle (broth should be 105°F or less so the miso's beneficial microflora and enzymes remain intact).

Add the miso broth to the soup in the pot.

Kendall's Tasty Tip: I slurped down a lot of miso soup while undergoing chemo. I felt it gave me such strength and energy. It was often the perfect meal on chemo days, or the day or two after when I was still feeling nauseous, weak and tired.

Sweet and Creamy Tomato Soup

brain boosting | comfort food | dehydration defending | mood balancing | vegan | vegetarian

This soup is a go-to recipe for us when we have a craving for something sweet and creamy. We almost can't stop eating it—it's that good! Tomatoes and butternut squash offer lots of carotenoid-fueled cancer-kicking power. The principle fatty acid in coconut milk is lauric acid, which is the same fat found in mother's milk and is known to support brain development and contribute to healthy bones.

Yield: makes 10 cups

1 tablespoon olive oil

1 large onion, coarsely chopped

2 teaspoons sea salt, divided

3 garlic cloves, minced

1 (2 to 2½ pound) butternut squash, seeded and cubed

4 large tomatoes, coarsely chopped (about 4 cups)

1 can coconut milk (13.5 to 14 ounces)

2 cups Vegetable Stock (page 271) or store-bought

½ cup fresh cilantro, chopped

In a stockpot, heat the olive oil over medium heat. Add the onion, sprinkle with a teaspoon of the sea salt, and sauté for about five minutes. Then add the garlic, another teaspoon of the sea salt, and continue sautéing for another one to two minutes, stirring so the garlic doesn't burn.

Add the squash, tomatoes, coconut milk and vegetable broth. Bring to a boil then reduce heat to low and simmer, covered, for about forty-five minutes or until squash is very tender. Remove from heat, add cilantro if desired and purée using a handheld immersion blender.

Annette's Tasty Tip: No need to be worried about coconut's saturated fat. Coconut has important anticarcinogenic, antipathogenic, antiviral, antifungal and antimicrobial properties (whew!) and the fat content (or oil) within the coconut has been shown to help support weight loss.

Satisfying Split Pea Soup

constipation kicking | comfort food | dehydration defending |
fatigue fighting and adrenal support | mouth sore friendly | vegan | vegetarian

There's something about split pea soup that makes us feel all warm and cozy and satisfied. Our recipe provides lots of creamy goodness, with plenty of protein, fiber and veggies to boot. It's like a food version of a snuggie. Packaged split peas can be found where the grains and beans are in your grocery store. Store them in an airtight container, with a bay leaf added for freshness.

Yield: makes 10 cups

2 tablespoons olive oil

2 large onions, coarsely chopped (about 3½ cups)

3 teaspoons sea salt, divided

2 large carrots, large dice (about ¾ cup)

4 celery ribs, large dice (about 1¾ cups)

2 teaspoons ground cumin

½ teaspoon freshly ground black pepper

8 cups Vegetable Stock (page 271) or store-bought

2 cups green or yellow split peas, soaked

2 bay leaves

1 tablespoon fresh or dried dill, minced

Heat the olive oil in a stockpot over medium-high heat then sauté the onions along with a teaspoon of sea salt for ten minutes. Add the carrots, celery, cumin, one teaspoon of the salt and pepper and sauté another five minutes. Next add the vegetable broth, split peas, remaining teaspoon of sea salt and bay leaves. Bring to a boil and then reduce heat to low, simmering for about two and a half hours or until the split peas are soft. Adjust seasonings, remove bay leaves and purée using a handheld immersion blender. Add the dill before serving.

Annette's Tasty Tip: To speed up cooking time and enhance digestibility, the split peas should be placed in a bowl, covered with water and soaked overnight. Drain and rinse before using in the recipe.

Smoky Squash Soup

dehydration defending | immune boosting | vegan | vegetarian

Kabocha (kah-BOH-cha) squash is a hard winter squash with a dull, bumpy, dark green shell that is originally from Japan. Kabocha has bright orange flesh, due to its high level of caratenoids. Low in calories, high in nutrients and fiber, there's a lot to love about this sweet veggie. Instead of pepitas, you can also use the kabocha's seeds. Depending on the variety of smoked paprika you use, you may have to adjust the spice level to your taste.

Yield: makes 6½ cups

1 large onion, thinly sliced

3 garlic cloves, minced

1 tablespoon olive oil

2 teaspoons smoked paprika

3 tablespoons apple juice

2 pounds kabocha or other winter squash, seeded and cubed

3½ cups Vegetable Stock (page 271) or store-bought

2 bay leaves

Sea salt and freshly ground black pepper

Pepitas for garnish

Add the onion and garlic to the cold oil in a stockpot then place over medium-high heat and sauté for ten minutes. Add the smoked paprika and sauté for an additional minute. Deglaze the stockpot by adding the apple juice and stirring. Add the squash, vegetable stock and bay leaves and simmer until the squash is tender, about thirty minutes. Remove from the heat, discard the bay leaves, and purée using a handheld immersion blender. Season the soup with salt and pepper and sprinkle the pepitas into each bowlful before serving.

Annette's Tasty Tip: Pepitas, or pumpkin seeds, are a delicious source of phosphorus, magnesium, manganese, zinc and iron as well as a good source of protein. Purchase raw pepitas then pan-toast them in a dry skillet (we love cast iron!) over low heat, stirring frequently. Toss them onto soups, add to salads or trail mix, or just munch on them as a healthy snack.

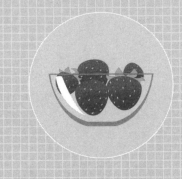

Snack Time

Crispy Kale Chips

blood boosting | detoxifying | hormone balancing | immune boosting | vegan | vegetarian

If you aren't familiar with kale, these chips are a fantastic, super tasty way to try it. They are addicting! The recipe helps you to put more powerful cancer-kicking kale into your diet—and might even satisfy a chip craving in the process! Kids love to munch on these, too, and don't even realize they're eating their veggies!

Yield: makes 4 cups

5 large kales leaves, stems removed, torn into chip-size portions

1 tablespoon olive oil

2 teaspoons nutritional yeast

Sea salt

Preheat the oven to 350°F.

Rinse and completely dry the kale, using a salad spinner then a dry towel. Place the kale in a bowl and toss with the olive oil, yeast and salt. Spread the kale in a thin layer on a cookie sheet lined with parchment paper, and bake for twelve to fifteen minutes or until the leaves are crisp. Check carefully near the end of the baking time to catch the kale chips when they are crisp and crackly, but before they turn too brown. Remove the cookie sheet from the oven and let the chips cool to room temperature.

Kendall's Tasty Tip: Try adding other seasonings to the chips as well. You can give them a kick with some cayenne pepper, or add a little tamari or a sprinkle of chopped chives. They are also yummy with ground pepper and garlic powder!

Fruity Salad

brain boosting | dehydration defending | detoxifying | mood balancing |
raw | vegan | vegetarian

Fruits are chockfull of vitamins, minerals and phytochemicals that fight back against cancer. Enjoy whole fruit to get the fiber as well, which slows digestion and the rate at which blood sugar rises. Fruit is an excellent, real-food way to satisfy a sweet craving nutritiously. When you are going through cancer treatment, it is generally fine to enjoy some fruit, but place a priority on vegetables in your diet.

Yield: makes about 3 cups

Pomegranate seeds from one pomegranate

½ cup pineapple chunks

1 cup fresh mixed berries (try raspberry, blackberry, strawberry, or blueberry)

1 medium carrot, shredded

¼ cup raw walnuts, chopped

¼ cup dried coconut, shredded and unsweetened

Cut the pomegranate in half and scoop the seeds out into a bowl half full with water. The pomegranate's white flesh will float and the seeds will sink. Scoop out and discard the white flesh, drain the water then add the seeds to a salad bowl. Add all the other ingredients, toss and serve.

Kendall's Tasty Tip: Pineapple contains the enzyme bromelain, which is helpful for reducing swelling and inflammation, especially after surgery. If you have mouth sores from chemotherapy, however, it's best to avoid it.

Potato Bruschetta Bites

comfort food | nausea nixing | vegan | vegetarian

When we were going through treatment, both of us often craved carb-dense comfort food. Potatoes were frequently a favorite. Here is a good way to satisfy that craving while upping the nutritional ante. By keeping the spud skin (rather than peeling it away), you also keep all the potato's nutrients and fiber. If Swiss chard is unavailable, try using baby spinach—or both! Adding veggie toppings and a drizzle of tasty omega-3 rich flax oil will make this tasty treat even more of a healthy bite.

Yield: makes 16 small potato bites

8 small red or golden potatoes, skins on

1½ teaspoons olive oil, divided

2 large Swiss chard leaves

½ small yellow onion

1 small tomato

½ bell pepper (red, yellow, or orange)

Fresh basil leaves

½ teaspoon garlic powder

¼ teaspoon salt

Dash of freshly ground black pepper

1 tablespoon flax oil

Preheat the oven to 375°F.

Scrub and rinse the potatoes well and cut each in half. Then slice about an eighth of an inch off the outside, rounded edge of each potato half, to keep the potato halves from wobbling. Place them, skin-side down, on a baking sheet lightly covered with ½ teaspoon of the olive oil. Bake for twenty-five minutes.

While the potatoes are baking, remove the stems of the Swiss chard and finely chop the leaves. Finely chop the onion, tomato, pepper and basil leaves and place in a small bowl with remaining olive oil. Add the garlic powder, salt and pepper and mix well until the vegetables are coated with oil. Remove the potatoes from the oven and top each with a spoonful of the chard mixture. Place them back in the oven for ten to fifteen minutes or until the potatoes can be easily pierced with a fork. Drizzle a little flax oil over each potato before serving.

Annette's Tasty Tip: In order to preserve its nutritional qualities, flax seed oil should not be used for cooking. Instead, add it to raw or already cooked foods.

Edamame Hummus

fatigue fighting and adrenal support | hormone balancing | vegan | vegetarian

This recipe provides a new way to enjoy edamame, and makes a unique hummus. It's great for snacking on when you want to keep your strength up, or need smaller protein-dense snacks between meals. The hummus keeps in the fridge for several days and can be used as a dip with everything from raw veggies to pita chips. Buy the edamame, frozen and blanched, in the freezer section of your grocery store and prepare them according to the package directions (usually boiling in water for about five minutes), and then use in creating this tasty snack.

Yield: makes about 1 cup

2 teaspoons extra-virgin olive oil

¼ teaspoon salt

¼ teaspoon ground coriander

½ teaspoon ground cumin

2 garlic cloves, finely chopped

1 cup edamame, prepared
(see preparation note, above)

⅓ cup fresh parsley

2 tablespoons tahini

3 tablespoons water

2 tablespoons lemon juice

Place all ingredients in a food processor and process until smooth, about one minute.

Kendall's Tasty Tip: It is always good to be mindful of your eating. But when you are going through cancer treatment and are challenged with keeping your weight at a healthy norm due to excessive weight loss, eating snacks can be important. Keep snacks that you love nearby so you can engage in some beneficial, "mindless" munching and get the calories you need, along with the right nutrients.

Triple Berry Popsicles

brain boosting | dehydration defending | mouth sore friendly |
nausea nixing | vegetarian

Strawberries are nutritional powerhouses. They have one of the highest levels of antioxidants to be found in commonly eaten foods, as well as the ability when consumed frequently to help keep inflammation markers in check. The fiber found in these whole fruits supports healthy intestinal function and helps balance blood sugar levels. And guess what? Making and eating popsicles is just as fun now as it was when you were a kid! If fresh berries are not available, reach for frozen, then thaw your berries before blending.

Yield: makes 4 popsicles

¾ cup strawberries, stems removed

½ cup blueberries

¼ cup red raspberries

3 tablespoons unfiltered apple juice

1½ tablespoons honey, optional

Combine the berries and juice in a blender and process until smooth, about one minute. Taste then add honey if desired. Pour mixture into four popsicle molds, inserting sticks. Freeze until solid, about three hours.

Annette's Tasty Tip: This is a snack your child can help you make, or your teen can make for you. These are perfect for warm days and sore, dry mouths. Somehow, enjoying a popsicle can give you the feeling of being young and carefree—pure, good-for-you indulgence.

Herbed Popcorn

comfort food | constipation kicking | vegan | vegetarian

Add a nutritional punch to your munch by skipping the standard butter-and-salt popcorn routine and instead go for herbs and spices. They add not only exciting, new flavor but also contribute a host of cancer-kicking qualities!

Yield: makes about 8 cups

2 tablespoons olive oil

¼ cup popcorn kernels

1 teaspoon dried dill

1 teaspoon nutritional yeast

¼ teaspoon sea salt

Additional toppings, if desired:

Rosemary

Thyme

Oregano

Garlic powder

Ground cumin

Ground coriander

Place the oil in a large heavy pot with a handle and add the corn kernels. Heat over medium-high heat, covered, occasionally shaking the pot back and forth. When the popping slows inside the pot, remove it from heat and place popcorn in a large bowl. Top immediately with the dill, nutritional yeast and salt. If desired, add additional herb toppings.

Annette's Tasty Tip: Popcorn was a food I craved during treatment and was easy to keep nearby and munch on whenever I needed a snack. Make a larger portion and store in an airtight container for use throughout the week and to take along when out and about.

Tasty Trail Mix

brain boosting | fatigue fighting and adrenal support |
immune boosting | vegan | vegetarian

Nuts provide healthy fats along with important minerals. When looking for nutritionally dense high-calorie food to keep weight on during treatment, this trail-mix snack makes a smart choice. You can choose roasted nuts if you need to avoid raw foods. If weight gain is a concern, nuts and seeds can still be enjoyed in moderation.

Yield: makes 2½ cups

½ cup raw almonds

½ cup raw cashews

½ cup raw sunflower seeds

¼ cup raisins

¼ cup dried cranberries

¼ cup dark-chocolate chips

¼ cup raw pecans

1 tablespoon sesame seeds

⅛ cup coconut flakes, unsweetened

¼ cup raw pepitas

Combine all ingredients and enjoy!

Kendall's Tasty Tip: I kept baggies of this trail mix made up, to grab when I was on the way to a treatment session or when I knew I would be out of the house for a while and wanted to avoid vending-machine food.

Coconut Goji Energy Bars

fatigue fighting and adrenal support | hormone balancing | immune boosting |
mood balancing | vegan | vegetarian

When you are looking for a nutrient-dense snack at home or on the go, but don't want to depend on what someone else packaged into the energy bars at your supermarket, make your own! It's easy, more economical, and you can customize it, too. Here's our recipe for energy bars with some of our favorite superfood ingredients including coconut, cacao, goji berries, chia seeds and maca. They are all immune-system boosting, energy giving, mood and weight balancing and—let's not forget—delicious.

Yield: makes 9 3-by-3 inch squares

2 cups raw almonds

2 cups dried coconut, shredded and unsweetened

4 vanilla beans, split lengthwise, insides scraped

3 tablespoons raw cacao nibs

2 tablespoons goji berries, finely chopped

2 teaspoons maca powder

2 pinches sea salt

¼ cup unrefined coconut oil, melted

½ cup brown-rice syrup

1 tablespoon chia seeds

Place the almonds in a food processor or blender and process until ground. In a large bowl combine the ground almonds with the coconut, vanilla bean seeds, cacao nibs, goji berries, maca and sea salt. Mix well. Drizzle the coconut oil over the mixture and stir well. Then add the brown-rice syrup and combine thoroughly, using your hands if necessary.

Press the mixture into an 8-by-8-inch pan, using the back of a large spoon to the press mixture in firmly. Then scatter the chia seeds over the coconut mixture and press them in using the back of the spoon.

Place the pan in the refrigerator for a few hours or overnight. Remove and then cut into desired size. May be stored at room temperature.

Annette's Tasty Tip: Chia seeds, though tiny, pack a huge nutritional punch. They are a great source of protein, minerals, fiber and those healthy omega-3 fatty acids. Sprinkle them on porridge, yogurt, fruit salad and add them to baked goods and smoothies.

Lentil Spread

blood boosting | comfort food | constipation kicking | fatigue fighting and adrenal support | vegan | vegetarian

If you are like your Girlfriends, you're gonna love our lentil spread for its versatility and great taste. Use it as a dip with fresh veggies, toast some pita then use it as a spread, or roll up in a wrap with your favorite fixins for an easy and nutritious lunch on the go.

Yield: makes 3 cups

1 cup brown lentils

1 (1-inch) piece kombu

1 large onion, diced (about 2 cups)

4 garlic cloves, minced

½ cup sliced mushrooms

1 tablespoon Dijon mustard

¾ cup chopped walnuts, pan-toasted

1 tablespoon balsamic or rice vinegar

¼ cup fresh parsley, chopped

½ teaspoon sea salt

¼ teaspoon ground cumin

¼ teaspoon paprika

Rinse the lentils and place in a pot with three cups of water and the kombu, onion, garlic and mushrooms. Bring to a boil for ten minutes then cover and reduce heat to low, simmering for about forty minutes until the lentils are very tender and the water is absorbed. While the lentils are cooking, pan-toast the walnuts. Then remove the kombu from the lentils and combine the lentils, walnuts and all the remaining ingredients in a food processor. Pulse until well mixed and smooth.

Quick Veggies and Delish Dips

constipation kicking | *dehydration defending* | *detoxifying* | *immune boosting* |
mouth sore friendly | *vegan* | *vegetarian*

There's nothing like having an array of cancer-fighting veggies ready to munch on and at your fingertips through the day. Prep and cook once then eat for various snacks and meals. It's also an option to enjoy these veggies raw, though if you are immune-compromised, this quick-boil method is an easy alternative.

Quick Cook Veggies

Your choice of fresh vegetables: Try broccoli, cauliflower, kohlrabi, carrots, daikon, asparagus, rutabaga and fennel

Create an "assembly line" of veggies. Wash and prep the veggies so they are in bite-size pieces. Cut the broccoli and cauliflower into florets and stem spears; firm veggies such as daikon, kohlrabi and rutabaga can be cut into slices.

Fill a stockpot about a third of the way with water and bring to a boil. Set a large colander inside a large bowl next to the stockpot. When the water is at a full boil, place the first type of vegetable in the water and replace the lid on the pot, leaving the heat setting on high. In about two to three minutes the water should come back to a boil and the vegetables can be removed from the water using a slotted spoon then placed in the colander to drain. Replace the lid on the stockpot; wait a moment or two for the water to resume boiling. Repeat this process with the remaining vegetables, adjusting cooking times as dictated by vegetable size and thickness. The vegetables should be crisp when removed from the pot, not soft. After each vegetable has drained, remove it from the colander and place it in a glass storage container before straining the next vegetable. Eat immediately or store in the refrigerator to eat as a snack through the day either plain, with herbs and spices or using a dip, like one of ours in the recipes on the following page.

Creamy Bell Pepper Dip

immune boosting | raw | vegan | vegetarian

Yield: makes 1¼ cups

1 bell pepper, chopped
(red, orange, or yellow)

3 tablespoons extra-virgin olive oil

½ cup raw cashews

½ cup raw sunflower seeds

2 tablespoons lemon juice

½ teaspoon sea salt

Place all ingredients in a food processor or high-speed blender and pulse to combine until smooth. Add additional olive oil as desired for consistency.

Creamy Veggie Goodness Dip

fatigue fighting and adrenal support | hormone balancing | immune boosting | vegan | vegetarian

Yield: makes 1¼ cups

6 ounces extra-firm organic tofu

¼ cup sweet onion or scallions, diced

⅛ cup fresh parsley

1 kale leaf, stem removed

½ tablespoon garlic or chives, finely chopped

1 small carrot, grated

½ tablespoon prepared mustard

½ tablespoon real maple syrup

1 tablespoon lemon juice

½ tablespoon brown-rice vinegar

½ tablespoon white or yellow miso

1½ tablespoons extra-virgin olive oil

⅛ teaspoon sea salt

Place all ingredients in a food processor or high-speed blender and pulse to combine until smooth. Add water by the tablespoon as needed, to reach the desired consistency. Refrigerate for a few hours to allow flavors to mix before serving.

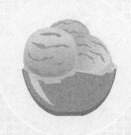

Sweetness

Berry Cobbler

comfort food | fatigue fighting and adrenal support | immune boosting | vegan | vegetarian

This cobbler is our healthier take on a traditional treat and contains antioxidant-rich, cancer-fighting berries. It has a nice crumbly topping and some serious sweet-berry flavor. We have to admit that sometimes we even enjoy a small piece with breakfast (if there's actually any left over from dessert).

Yield: makes one 10-by-7-inch pan

Fruit Filling:

5 cups fresh mixed berries, rinsed (if using strawberries, sliced in half)

2 tablespoons arrowroot powder

¼ cup maple-sugar granules

½ teaspoon ground cinnamon

1 teaspoon vanilla extract

Topping:

1 cup rolled oats

½ cup spelt flour or whole-wheat pastry flour

¼ cup maple-sugar granules

¼ cup dried coconut, shredded and unsweetened

¼ cup softened unrefined coconut oil, melted, or avocado oil

½ cup chopped walnuts or almonds

⅛ teaspoon salt

Preheat the oven to 375°F.

Gently press the berries on paper towels, to dry off excess rinsing water. In a mixing bowl, combine the berries, arrowroot powder, maple-sugar granules, cinnamon and vanilla. Place berry mixture in a 10-by-7-inch pan.

Combine the topping ingredients in a mixing bowl and mix until crumbly. Spread the topping over the fruit, cover with foil and bake for twenty minutes. Remove the foil and bake for an additional fifteen to twenty minutes or until golden brown. Remove from the oven and cool for at least fifteen minutes before serving.

Chocolate-Raspberry Mousse

comfort food | fatigue fighting and adrenal support |
mood balancing | vegan | vegetarian

The awesome thing about tofu is that it takes on any flavor you combine it with. In this case, we're giving it a decadent chocolaty-raspberry taste. This mousse will practically melt in your mouth, and you'll never know it's made with tofu. This recipe also uses maple syrup for sweetening, which is a better choice than refined white sugar—just make sure you get the real stuff and not "pancake syrup," which often contains other ingredients like corn syrup and sometimes no real maple syrup at all.

Yield: makes 2½ cups

1 pound silken tofu

1 cup raspberries, fresh or frozen

½ cup raw cacao powder

½ cup real maple syrup

Process the tofu in a food processor for one minute, or until smooth. Add the raspberries, cacao powder and maple syrup and process for thirty seconds, or until well combined. Store the mousse in the refrigerator until you're ready to serve it.

Kendall's Tasty Tip: This is the perfect dessert to eat with your gal pals. Ask them to come over and make you a healthy dinner, and let them know you'll reward them afterward with this mousse.

Key-Lime Custard Pie

comfort food | fatigue fighting and adrenal support | vegan | vegetarian

Kendall: One of my favorite desserts growing up was Key lime pie, and I am psyched to say that this healthier, dairy-free and less-refined version is freakin' fantastic! The nuts in the custard and crust are full of protein and make it rather filling, so you really only need a small slice to satisfy your sweet-and-sour craving. And yeah, you should probably avoid this tangy dessert if you are dealing with mouth sores.

Yield: makes 8 pie slices

Crust:

½ cup raw almonds

½ cup pepitas (pumpkin seeds)

1 teaspoon unrefined coconut oil, melted

1 tablespoon real maple syrup

¼ teaspoon salt

Pie Filling:

1½ cups raw cashews

¾ cup coconut milk

⅓ cup unrefined coconut oil, melted

¾ cup lime juice

¾ cup real maple syrup

½ teaspoon lime zest

½ teaspoon lemon zest

Mix the crust ingredients in a food processor for one minute or until they are ground into crust dough. Use your fingers to firmly press the dough into a pie plate.

To make the pie filling, first add the cashews to the food processor and process for one minute until finely ground. Add the coconut milk, coconut oil, lime juice, maple syrup, lime and lemon zest and process one to two minutes or until smooth. Scoop the pie filling into the crust; use a spoon to spread evenly. Refrigerate for two hours or overnight. Remove from the refrigerator and let the pie sit at room temperature for five to ten minutes to soften slightly before serving.

No-Bake Oatmeal Raisin Balls

comfort food | fatigue fighting and adrenal support | raw | vegan | vegetarian

Just the smell of these treats will have you feeling all snuggly. In this recipe you'll also get a boost to your mood—and your health!—from cinnamon. And these couldn't be easier to make. Just a few ingredients, no oven time and viola: instant comfort. No refined sugars to cause a blood sugar crash; the sweetness comes instead from a whole food—dates! Experiment with various types of dates, like Medjool, Deglet Noor or Zahidi, for different flavors.

Yield: makes 18 to 20 small balls

1 cup dates, pitted

1¾ cups rolled oats

2 teaspoons ground cinnamon

1 teaspoon chia seeds

¾ cup raisins

Soak the dates in filtered water for ten minutes. Drain off the water.

Combine the oats, cinnamon, dates and chia seeds in a food processor then process until the ingredients stick together, forming a "dough." If the dough mixture doesn't stick together well, add one to two teaspoons of filtered water. Add the raisins and process until combined. Use your fingers to press the dough into small balls for serving. Store balls in the refrigerator, covered, for up to ten days.

Annette's Tasty Tip: These treats are fantastic to have nearby when you need a small bite to eat or when you are on the go and want a healthy snack to take along.

Chocolate-Chip
Peanut Butter Cookies

comfort food | fatigue fighting and adrenal support | mood balancing | vegan | vegetarian

If you're used to cookies made with refined white flour, you will likely find these to be a little richer, which means you'll only need one or two to feel satisfied. Teff flour has a chocolaty, nutty flavor itself, so it is a perfect complement to this recipe. Teff is a tiny grass grain native to northeast Africa. It is naturally gluten-free and higher in protein than wheat flour. Teff is also a good source of fiber, calcium and plant-based iron. If you cannot find teff flour in your local store, you can order it online.

Yield: makes 2 dozen cookies

1¼ cup peanut butter

⅔ cup real maple syrup

½ cup plain, unsweetened applesauce

1 tablespoon vanilla extract

1½ cups teff flour

¾ cup dark-chocolate chips

Preheat the oven to 350°F.

Combine the peanut butter, maple syrup, applesauce and vanilla using a mixer or food processor. Add the teff flour and then stir in the chocolate chips to form a dough. Shape the dough into small balls and flatten them gently with the back of a spoon or fingers onto an ungreased cookie sheet. Bake them for about fifteen minutes, then transfer to a cooling rack.

Annette's Tasty Tip: This recipe is a favorite when I am longing for a cookie but want to make it a healthy treat. They freeze fine as well, so you can remove and thaw as needed.

Chocolate-Cherry Fudge Brownies

comfort food | constipation kicking | fatigue fighting and adrenal support | mood balancing | mouth sore friendly | vegan | vegetarian

These brownies are made with black beans instead of flour, so you get plenty of protein, fiber and extra nutrients. The oats and pecans add even more vitamins and minerals, so you enjoy a chocolaty, decadent dessert that is nutritious. Create a flax egg by whisking together one tablespoon ground flax seeds with three tablespoons of lukewarm water for each egg needed. Allow to sit for five minutes before using in the recipe.

Yield: makes sixteen 2-inch brownies

1 package organic dark-chocolate or vegan chocolate chips (12 ounces)

3 tablespoons unrefined coconut oil, plus additional for greasing

1 can organic black beans, drained and rinsed (15 ounces)

3 flax eggs (or organic, pastured eggs)

½ cup real maple syrup

½ cup organic rolled oats

2 teaspoons baking powder

½ cup pecans, finely chopped

¼ cup dried cherries, small dice

Preheat oven to 350°F. Lightly grease a 9-by-9 inch pan with coconut oil.

Place the chocolate chips and three tablespoons of the coconut oil in a heat-resistant glass container in a pot of water on medium heat. Heat until melted, stirring occasionally.

Transfer the melted chocolate mixture to a blender or food processor. Add all the remaining ingredients except the pecans and cherries and blend them until smooth, scraping sides as needed. Stir in the pecans and cherries. Pour batter into the prepared pan.

Bake for approximately fifty minutes (thirty or thirty-five minutes if using regular eggs) or until a toothpick inserted in the middle of the dish comes out mostly clean. Allow the brownies to sit then serve for a warm, gooey brownie, or place them in the refrigerator for several hours or overnight before serving, to create a firm, fudgy brownie.

Annette's Tasty Tip: Be sure to try with a scoop of our Coconut Ice Kreme with Cherry Swirl (see the next recipe) on top.

Coconut Ice Kreme
with Cherry Swirl

comfort food | mood balancing | mouth sore friendly | nausea nixing | vegan | vegetarian

Coconut milk creates this delicious, creamy, good-for-you ice kreme that's easy to make and hard to resist. Now you can enjoy your dessert without the dairy, the highly processed sugars and other unpronounceables that are in traditional ice cream.

Yield: makes 6 cups

Ice Kreme:

3 cups coconut milk (not light)

¼ cup sucanat

2 vanilla beans, split lengthwise with insides scraped, or 1 tablespoon vanilla extract

¼ cup dried coconut, shredded and unsweetened

Cherry Swirl:

½ cup sweet cherries, frozen

2 tablespoons real maple syrup

Combine all the ice kreme ingredients and place the mixture in a 13-by-9-inch glass dish in the freezer, stirring every thirty minutes until firm, about two hours.

Combine the cherry swirl ingredients in a blender or food processor.

Add the cherry mixture by gently swirling it through the ice kreme using a spoon. Freeze for an additional half an hour. Allow ice kreme to soften at room temperature for fifteen to thirty minutes before serving.

Pumpkin Loaf with Maple Glaze

comfort food | immune boosting | mood balancing | mouth sore friendly | vegan | vegetarian

We love it when we can have our cake—or loaf, as in this case—and eat it, too. We can tell you about all the amazing ingredients in this recipe, like hemp milk, flax seeds, spices, nuts and pumpkin. Or we can just tell you that this pumpkin loaf is moist, satisfying and dessert- and snack-worthy. Either way, you'll love it for its nutritional goodness and comfort-food yumminess.

Yield: makes 1 loaf

Coconut oil

1 cup hemp milk or other nondairy milk

1 tablespoon ground flax seeds

2½ cups spelt flour

1½ teaspoons baking powder

2 teaspoons baking soda

¼ teaspoon sea salt

3 teaspoons ground cinnamon

½ teaspoon allspice

¼ teaspoon ground nutmeg

½ teaspoon ground gingerroot

⅓ cup applesauce

½ banana, very ripe, mashed

1 tablespoon apple cider vinegar

½ cup sucanat

2 teaspoons vanilla extract

2 cups pumpkin purée
(or one 15-ounce can)

¼ cup raw walnuts or pecans, chopped

¼ cup raisins

Preheat the oven to 350°F. Lightly grease a 9-by-5-inch loaf pan using coconut oil.

Warm the hemp milk in a small saucepan. Remove from heat and add the ground flax seeds. Allow to sit for at least five minutes.

In a large mixing bowl, stir together the flour, baking powder, baking soda, salt and spices. Add the milk-flax mixture, applesauce, banana, vinegar, sucanat and vanilla. Stir to combine. Fold in the pumpkin then the nuts and the raisins.

Pour the batter into the loaf pan and bake for seventy minutes or until a toothpick pierced into the center of the loaf comes out clean. Allow the loaf to cool in the pan on a wire rack for fifteen minutes before removing it from the pan. Cool it completely, adding the maple glaze if desired and then slice to serve.

Maple Glaze

We love the pumpkin loaf straight up, or with a dollop of apple butter spread over a slice. For those of you who need a little extra sweetness, here's a glaze for a special occasion.

⅓ cup organic powdered sugar
2 tablespoons real maple syrup
1 teaspoon vanilla extract

Whisk the ingredients together, and drizzle over the cooled loaf.

Kendall's Tasty Tip: The sucanat used in the pumpkin loaf is a minimally processed form of cane sugar. Sugar cane is crushed, the juice is extracted, heated then cooled. Sucanat retains the molasses, including the minerals it contains, which gives it a complex flavor and makes it much more of a whole food than refined sugar.

Green Tea-Mango Sorbet

*brain boosting | dehydration defending | mood balancing |
mouth sore friendly | vegan | vegetarian*

Who says you can only drink your green tea? Here's a delicious way to get more of the cancer-kicking power of green tea into your life, including your dessert. The mangoes are a excellent source of vitamin C and antioxidants.

Yield: makes about 2 cups

1 cup water

⅓ cup loose green-tea leaves

⅓ cup brown-rice syrup

2 cups mangoes, frozen, chopped

Lime zest (optional)

Heat the water in a saucepan; remove it from the heat just before it comes to a boil. Add the tea leaves (a tea infuser is best; otherwise toss in the leaves then remove with a strainer after steeping). Steep for five minutes then remove leaves but do not press them. Add the brown-rice syrup to the tea and stir to dissolve. Allow the tea to cool.

Combine the tea mixture and the mangoes in a blender; blend at high speed until smooth. Serve immediately for a soft-serve texture. For a more solid texture, scoop it into a container and freeze for an hour or more. Remove from the freezer and allow to soften briefly to ease scooping.

Annette's Tasty Tip: You can get even more green-tea goodness into your diet by cooking with it as well. Make a pot of tea then reserve some to drink and use the rest as part of the liquid when cooking your grains or beans.

Juicy Jello

comfort food | dehydration defending | mood balancing | mouth sore friendly | nausea nixing | vegan | vegetarian

We don't know about you, but your Girlfriends don't think jello should just be for the 12-and-under set. Give us some of this juicy jello any day and we feel all young and care-free again. This recipe is a cinch to make and perfect for a warm summer day, or when you need something that goes down easy. Problem is, you're not going to want to share with your kids!

Yield: makes nine 3-by-3-inch squares

3 cups fruit juice (a single juice, such as apple, or a combination of juices such as blueberry-pomegranate)

¼ cup brown-rice syrup

3 teaspoons agar-agar

½ cup fresh fruit, in bite-size pieces

Combine all the ingredients except the fresh fruit in a pot and slowly bring to a boil, stirring often, for about ten minutes. Allow to boil for a few seconds, then reduce heat and simmer, stirring constantly and watching for agar-agar flakes to dissolve, about five minutes.

Transfer to a 9-by-9-inch glass casserole, gently add the fruit pieces, and place in the refrigerator for one hour or until firm.

Cut into pieces and serve.

Annette's Tasty Tip: Agar-agar is a tasteless sea veggie, so you get all the cancer-kicking power of sea vegetables in this delicious dessert without any of the gelatin, refined sugar and artificial junk in the store-bought Jello box.

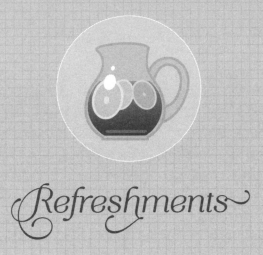

Refreshments

Blueberry Lemonade

dehydration defending | detoxifying | immune boosting | raw |
respiratory-system support | vegan | vegetarian

Enjoy this refreshing lemonade on hot days or when you need a hydrating pick-me-up. Blueberries offer antioxidant cancer-fighting power, along with lots of vitamin C to boost your immune system. Lemons promote immunity and help fight off infection, and because they are alkalizing, they help to balance the body's pH. Be cautious about drinking this if you are suffering from chemo-induced heartburn or mouth sores: It can aggravate either condition.

Yield: makes 20 ounces

Juice from 2 medium lemons (⅓ cup)

¾ cup frozen blueberries

1½ cups water

2 tablespoons real maple syrup

Add all the ingredients to a blender and mix until smooth. If you are using fresh blueberries, add a few cubes of ice to the blender then blend before serving.

Annette's Tasty Tip: In the summertime, I pour my blueberry lemonade in a nice glass and add a straw and little paper umbrella. Then I head outdoors to my lounge chair and enjoy some sunshine.

Carrot-Beet Juice

blood boosting | dehydration defending | detoxifying | fatigue fighting and adrenal support | immune boosting | mood balancing | vegan | vegetarian

To make raw juice, we highly recommend using an electric juicer. If you don't have a juicer, you can use a high-powered blender and add some water when mixing the veggies. Then pour through a mesh strainer into a glass to collect the juice; discard the fibrous part of the fruit and vegetables. This juice combination offers sweetness with major blood and immune-boosting power.

Yield: makes about 10 ounces

1 carrot, roughly chopped

1 small beet, roughly chopped

2 apples, roughly chopped

½-inch piece gingerroot

Add all the ingredients to a juicer and collect the juice in a glass. Drink immediately, for the full energizing, nutrient-rich goodness.

Kendall's Tasty Tip: You may need to chop up your fruit and veggie portions larger or smaller, depending on your juicer. Just make sure the pieces are small enough to fit down its chute.

Krazy Kale Juice

We know: What?! Now you want me to drink my kale? But we think you'll be pleasantly surprised with this juice. The pear and apple help sweeten it up, and you'll love the pretty, bright green color. We highly recommend using a juicer, but a blender can also be used (see the previous recipe, Carrot-Beet Juice, for instructions).

Yield: makes 8 ounces

5 kale leaves

1 celery rib

1 pear

1 apple

Wash all the fruit and vegetables and chop roughly, leaving stems and seeds if desired. Add all the ingredients to a juicer and collect the juice in a glass. Drink immediately; fresh juice is healthiest straight from the juicer.

Watermelon Slushie

dehydration defending | immune boosting | mouth sore friendly |
nausea nixing | raw | vegan | vegetarian

This cooling treat is wonderful in the summertime and goes down easily when you're dealing with a sore mouth and throat or nausea. It's simple to make and is full of vitamins C, A, B1, B6 and magnesium. Watermelon also contains the electrolytes potassium and sodium, which can help to replenish your body after you've lost fluids. One more fabulous fact about watermelon: It is full of the antioxidant lycopene, which helps to neutralize free radicals and protect against cancer.

Yield: makes about 32 ounces

8 ice cubes

2½ cups watermelon, seedless or with seeds removed, cubed

Real maple syrup or honey to taste (optional)

Place the ice cubes in a blender and pulse on ice-crush setting. Add the cubed watermelon to the blender and pulse to mix. Add natural sweetener if desired before serving.

Annette's Tasty Tip: Watermelon was one food that I constantly craved during chemotherapy. I couldn't get enough of it! If you are dealing with chemo-induced menopause and the associated hot flashes, this watermelon slushie will help cool you down while keeping you hydrated.

Vital Greens Tea

blood boosting | dehydration defending | detoxifying | fatigue fighting and adrenal support |
immune boosting | mood balancing | respiratory-system support | vegetarian

This tea can be conveniently made from the stems of leafy greens that you are not using in cooking. We like to add in a few leaves, too. Save the stems in an airtight glass container in the fridge to make this tea within a couple of days, or brew the tea immediately. You get an amazing boost of calcium, iron, magnesium and plenty of other nutrients that will help strengthen your immune system, support your blood and organs, balance your hormones and moods, provide energy and aid in detoxifying your body. You may wish to alter the amount of greens or water to make this tea stronger or weaker.

Yield: makes 28 ounces

Stems from leafy greens, roughly chopped (about 2 cups)

2 kale leaves, roughly chopped (or substitute dandelion, collards, mustard, arugula)

1 teaspoon ground cinnamon

Honey, to taste

Cinnamon stick

Bring four cups of water, stems and leaves and cinnamon to a boil. Cover and reduce heat to simmer for ten minutes. Pour the tea through a strainer into a pot, to filter out the greens. Ladle into mugs, add honey to taste and garnish with a cinnamon stick.

Sweet Ginger Tea

constipation kicking | dehydration defending | detoxifying | mood balancing | nausea nixing | vegan | vegetarian

Ginger is a strong antioxidant and immune booster, so this is a perfect tea to drink for a cold or when fighting any disease. It has even been shown to suppress metastasis! Ginger is antimicrobial, antifungal and anti-inflammatory, and helps with nausea. The dates sweeten this tea, contain vital minerals such as iron, calcium and magnesium, and are a natural aid in easing constipation.

Yield: makes 64 ounces

3- to 4-inch piece of gingerroot

10 Medjool dates

Cut the gingerroot into three pieces, then smash with a mallet or rolling pin to release the flavor. Remove pits from the dates. Fill a pot with eight cups of water and add the ginger and dates. Bring to a boil, then reduce to simmer for thirty minutes. Strain the tea through a fine-mesh strainer before serving.

Kendall's Tasty Tip: Save any leftover tea in a glass jar and store in the refrigerator to drink as an iced tea, or mix with sparkling mineral water to create your own healthy ginger ale.

Cool Cucumber-Mint Water
with Raspberry Ice

dehydration defending | detoxifying | mouth sore friendly | raw | vegan | vegetarian

We love to dress up our water. Plain old water is good stuff, necessary for optimal health and, honestly, we drink a ton of it. Adding a little flavor and some pretty color from some sweet whole foods adds pizzazz to this life-sustaining liquid.

Yield: makes 8 ounces

6 fresh raspberries

2 cucumber slices

6 fresh mint leaves

6 to 8 ounces filtered or sparkling mineral water

Add two raspberries to each of three ice-cube sections and fill with water. Place in the freezer for several hours until frozen. In an eight- to twelve-ounce glass, place the cucumber slices, mint leaves and raspberry ice cubes. Add the filtered or sparkling water to top off the glass.

Annette's Tasty Tip: Mint is an herb that is easy to grow yourself. It can be used in many ways in the kitchen. One of our favorites is to use the fresh leaves to brew a calming and relaxing mint tea. Steep several sprigs in hot water for five minutes, grab a good book, strain the tea and enjoy.

Sunny Hemp Mylk

dehydration defending | fatigue fighting and adrenal support |
mouth sore friendly | vegan | vegetarian

This nutty-tasting mylk can be used in other recipes such as our smoothies, or just drink it by itself. It's also fantastic on our Nutty Cranberry-Coconut Granola (page 214). The hemp seeds are a significant source of magnesium, a mineral frequently lacking in diets in the U.S., and they are a vegetarian source of protein and omega-3s.

Yield: makes 40 ounces

½ cup raw sunflower seeds

½ cup raw hemp seeds, shelled

1 to 2 tablespoons real maple syrup

4 cups filtered water

Soak the sunflower seeds in water for four to five hours. Drain and rinse. Add the hemp seeds, soaked sunflower seeds and maple syrup to a blender with 2 cups of the filtered water. Blend for one minute, then add rest of the water and blend for another minute. This mylk can be stored in the refrigerator for three to four days.

Annette's Tasty Tip: If your blender does not blend the mylk enough for your liking, try pouring through a fine-mesh strainer, cheesecloth or nut-milk bag, before saving the liquid.

Citrus Spritzer

dehydration defending | fatigue fighting and adrenal support |
nausea nixing | raw | vegan | vegetarian

This is a simple, refreshing beverage that is packed with vitamin C. It also can help to balance the blood's pH, because lemons are alkalizing once they have been digested in the body. The carbonation can help to ease nausea. But if you are dealing with mouth sores, be wary of the citrus.

Yield: makes 44 ounces

1 small orange	Cut the orange, lemon and lime in half. Squeeze the juice from one half of each fruit into a pitcher. Add the sparkling mineral water. Cut the remaining halves of orange, lemon and lime into slices and add to the pitcher. Stir. Garnish each glass with a sprig of mint.
1 small lemon	
1 small lime	
5 cups sparkling mineral water	
Fresh mint sprigs	

Kendall's Tasty Tip: An easy way to flavor your water and keep it cool is to store sliced citrus in the freezer and add to your water or sparkling mineral water. Then you have flavored ice cubes!

Almond Mylk

constipation kicking | comfort food | dehydration defending | fatigue fighting and adrenal support | mouth sore friendly | raw | vegan | vegetarian

Some of our recipes call for almond milk, which you can purchase, or you can make your own. Making your own is easy and if you make it up ahead of time, it will keep in the refrigerator for three days. It tastes delicious in tea or coffee, in smoothies, cereals or in almost any recipe that calls for milk.

Yield: makes 20 ounces

1 cup raw almonds

2½ cups water

3 Medjool dates, pitted

¼ teaspoon ground cinnamon

Soak the almonds in cold water for eight hours or overnight. Drain and rinse. Add the almonds, water, dates and cinnamon to a high-powered blender and blend for two minutes at high speed. Strain the mixture through a nut-milk bag, cheesecloth or fine-mesh colander. Discard almond meal or save it for later use as a flour in baking.

Annette's Tasty Tip: If you can't find Medjool dates, just use what's available. If no dates are available, try adding a teaspoon of honey or maple syrup.

Resources

Below are some of the resources that may be helpful for those going through cancer or for anyone working on a cancer-kicking diet and lifestyle.

A SILVER LINING FOUNDATION (ASILVERLINIGFOUNDATION.ORG)
This foundation aids in obtaining dignified, respectful and equal access to quality cancer education and services for all. They work to ensure that socioeconomic status does not affect an individual's ability to obtain information, timely cancer screenings and diagnosis.

BLOG FOR A CURE (BLOGFORACURE.COM)
A cancer-blog community, where thousands of cancer survivors and loved ones blog about their experiences.

CANCERCARE (CANCERCARE.ORG)
CancerCare provides support services to individuals, families, caregivers and the bereaved to help them better cope with and manage the emotional and practical challenges arising from cancer. Their services, provided free of charge by professional oncology social workers, include counseling and support groups, educational publications and workshops, and financial assistance.

CANCER PLANNER (CANCER101.ORG)
CANCER101's mission is to empower cancer patients and their caregivers to take control over their diagnoses and engage them as active partners in their care, arming them with CANCER101 planners to navigate their cancer journey.

CANCER SCHMANCER (CANCERSCHMANCER.ORG)
This organization focuses on education, prevention and early detection of cancer, thereby eliminating mortality that can result from late-stage diagnosis. They aim to empower women to become medical consumers, to listen to their bodies, ask the right questions of their doctors and seek second opinions.

CARE PAGES (CAREPAGES.COM)

CarePages.com is an online community offering personalized Web sites where members facing a health challenge can relate their stories, post photos and update friends and family instantly. In turn, people who care send messages of love and encouragement.

CARING BRIDGE (CARINGBRIDGE.ORG)

This nonprofit offers free, personal and private websites to connect people experiencing a health challenge with family and friends.

CURE MAGAZINE (CURETODAY.COM)

Through the magazine Cure, educational forums, a resource guide for the newly diagnosed, books and a variety of online tools, CURE Media Group combines science and humanity to make cancer understandable.

FIGHT LIKE A GIRL (FIGHTLIKEAGIRLCLUB.COM)

This club was formed to provide a welcoming place where women (men are welcome, too!) battling cancer and other diseases, survivors, and loved ones can come together to share stories, experiences, hope and encouragement with one another.

FORCE—FACING OUR RISK OF CANCER EMPOWERED (FACINGOURRISK.ORG)

The only national nonprofit dedicated to improving the lives of individuals and families affected by hereditary breast and ovarian cancer.

FRIEND 4 LIFE (FRIEND4LIFE.ORG)

This organization helps persons recently diagnosed with cancer and their loved ones navigate the path through diagnosis, treatment and recovery by pairing them with a trained survivor with similar experiences, so they can face cancer with someone who's been there.

HEADCOVERS (HEADCOVERS.COM)

Headcovers has hats, turbans and wigs for hair loss available for purchase online.

I'M TOO YOUNG FOR THIS! CANCER FOUNDATION (STUPIDCANCER.COM)

Empowering young adults affected by cancer, this nonprofit organization offers age-appropriate support. They help to connect cancer peeps with young adult retreats, tweetups, happy hours and financial scholarships around the United States.

JILL'S LIST (JILLSLIST.COM)

Via a community of users, this site offers credible insights into the worlds of integrative, alternative and complementary medicine, while at the same time not losing sight of the importance of traditional medicine.

JUST IN TIME (SOFTHATS.COM)

This virtual company sells hats designed for women with hair loss. The collection includes hats, scarves, turbans and head wraps, and was started by a breast-cancer survivor.

LOCAL HARVEST (LOCALHARVEST.ORG)

Use this website to find farmers' markets, family farms, community-supported agriculture programs (CSAs) and other sources of sustainably grown food in your area. Some products, including produce, planting seeds, honey, teas and herbs are available for purchase through their online store.

LODGE CAST IRON (LODGEMFG.COM)

Shop online for American-made cast-iron cookware, such as Dutch ovens, skillets, country kettles and more.

LOTSA HELPING HANDS (LOTSAHELPINGHANDS.COM)

This site helps caregivers by giving their "circles of community" a way to help those going through cancer. Friends, neighbors and colleagues can create a free community website to help manage the daily tasks that become a challenge during times of need, and to keep everyone up to date on what's happening.

MEATLESS MONDAYS (MEATLESSMONDAYS.COM)

Meatless Monday is a nonprofit initiative of the Monday Campaigns, in association with the Johns Hopkins' Bloomberg School of Public Health, providing information and recipes to start each week with healthy, environmentally friendly, meat-free alternatives. Their goal is to help you reduce your meat consumption by 15 percent in order to improve your personal health and the health of the planet.

PLANET CANCER (PLANETCANCER.ORG)

Dedicated to the young-adult cancer community, Planet Cancer hosts the world's largest online community of young adults who have been affected by cancer. Planet Cancer also offers weekend retreats, and works to raise awareness and bring about positive change for young adults with cancer.

SHOP ORGANIC (SHOPORGANIC.COM)

Purchase organic groceries and goods from their website and have the order shipped to your door. Bulk, vegan, raw and gluten-free products available.

TALKABOUTHEALTH (TALKABOUTHEALTH.COM)

TalkAboutHealth is working to improve and personalize patient education and support. They offer patients and caregivers personalized, helpful and accurate health answers and support from leading medical professionals and trained peer survivors.

THE BEAUBEAU (4WOMEN.COM)

The BeauBeau® scarf is a fashionable alternative to a wig and is available in a variety of colors, prints and fabrics. The owner comes from a family with three generations of breast-cancer survivors, and she herself suffers from Alopecia Areata, sudden unexpected hair loss.

THINK BEFORE YOU PINK (THINKBEFOREYOUPINK.ORG)

Think Before You Pink, a project of Breast Cancer Action, was launched in response to the growing concern about the number of pink ribbon products on the market. The campaign calls for more transparency and accountability from companies that take part in breast-cancer fund-raising, and encourages consumers to ask critical questions about pink-ribbon promotions.

WELL SPOUSE ASSOCIATION (WELLSPOUSE.ORG)

The Well Spouse Association advocates for and addresses the needs of individuals caring for a chronically ill or disabled spouse or partner. They offer peer-to-peer support and educate health care professionals and the general public about the special challenges and unique issues "well" spouses face every day.

YOUNG SURVIVAL COALITION (YOUNGSURVIVAL.ORG)

Young Survival Coalition (YSC) is the premier global organization dedicated to the critical issues unique to young women who are diagnosed with breast cancer.

Acknowledgments

We began this journey with an idea and an intention: to bring friendship, provide support and share all we have learned on our cancer journeys with others so that their path might be just a bit easier. We are so very grateful to all of those who have played a part in making this happen. Thank you to Victoria Moran who helped us set out on the publishing path and offered her selfless time, care and support. To our agent, Matthew Carnicelli who has believed in this project and in us from the beginning: We thank him for his trust and for enabling us to be placed with such a great publishing house. Our editor, Jennifer Kasius, whose "yes" changed our lives, has championed this book from the get-go. We're so very grateful for her unconditional support and enthusiasm. We also thank Frances Soo Ping Chow, Seta Zink, Craig Herman, the sales staff and everyone at Running Press and Perseus Books for their dedication to creating a beautiful book out of our manuscript and getting it into the hands of our readers.

We'd like to thank Steve Legato, Debbie Whetstone Wahl and Mariellen Melker for an amazing photo shoot and the beautiful images of our recipes which now grace this book. We're also indebted to Steve for his generosity in filming and creating the trailer for our book. Many thanks as well to Johanna Jacobsen who graciously allowed her gorgeous music to be used in our trailer.

Mounds of gratitude to Christina Pirello who has been our wise mentor and constant champion: Your friendship and support is a priceless gift.

We met and studied at the Institute for Integrative Nutrition and are so thankful for Joshua Rosenthal and all of our teachers.

To the brilliant, kind and magnanimous Dr. David Katz, we bow in deep gratitude and respect. Thank you!

Annette:

I APPRECIATE MY husband Axel and my daughter Pearl more than words can express. Their steadfast presence, unwavering support and unconditional love and caring for me are priceless gifts. Axel's parents, especially my mother-in-law Rosi, have been a huge support, spending months with me as I recovered from surgeries and dealt with cancer treatments. I am so grateful for them.

I thank my co-author Kendall Scott, and am inspired by her strength, courage, and willingness to step off the beaten path with me and trust that the way would open for this book to be birthed through us. It has been an amazing ride and I am so happy we did it together.

I was blessed to have many friends supporting me throughout my cancer journeys as well as during the creation of the book. Thank you Christine, Griselda, Jen, Tammy, Su, Rodi, Tara, Eileen, Beth, Heather, Lynn, Anja, Amy, Dara, Sandy, Lis, Dorle, Diane, Gisela, Georganne, June, Joy, Jeanette, Rebecca, Robin, Sarah, Lisa, Sheri, Joanne, Marcy, Susan, Michelle, Stephanie, Charles and Jamie.

I met my tribe and blossomed into my new life at the Institute for Integrative Nutrition. My life is forever enriched by the friendships of Marie, Jalene, James, Jolene, Annette, Petra, Kendall, Meghan, Becca, Sam, Melissa, Diane, Meg, Lissa.

I am so thankful for the amazing team of doctors who have cared for me. Thank you Dr. Susan Domchek (with Robin Herzog and Trisha Garretson), Dr. Andrew Ashikari, Dr. Marcia Boraas, Dr. Andrew Salzberg, Dr. Thomas Randall (with Rebecca Kagan), Dr. Michael Reece ND, Dr. Stephen Rubin, Dr. Birgit Rakel, Dr. Steve Rosenzweig. I am also grateful for the many nurses who have cared for me. Special thanks to the nurses at the Rena Rowan Breast Center.

Mountains of gratitude for the practitioners and healers I have also had the privilege of working with, many of whom have become my dear friends. Thank you Jen Merritt, Petra Rakebrandt, Steph McCreary, Jesse Torgerson, Dory Ellen Fish,

Lauren Buckley, Rachel Weiss and Cara Frank.

I am truly privileged to work with amazing individuals and join them as a holistic health coach on their journeys to greater health and wellness. I appreciate my clients and all of the joy and purpose they bring into my life.

As with any list which tries to condense a lifetime into a few lines, this list is not complete. To all those whose lives have touched mine, whether they have brought me joy or pain (or both), I bow deeply to all as my teacher.

May all beings everywhere know peace.

Kendall:

TO MY PARTNER in life and love: Thank you, Tom, for always believing in me and making me laugh when I need to most. To my little love, Brogan: Thank you for bringing such joy and sweet smiles to my life and for your patience with your busy momma during the writing of this book.

For your love and support, through cancer and beyond, my deepest gratitude goes to: Mom and Dad, Lacey and Zac, Mary and Dick and the extended Scott clan, dear girlfriends Lindsey, Angie, Abby, Amanda, Stacie, Sarah and so many shining stars who offered love, light and prayers during tough times.

To "the guys": Tom, James, Matt, Joe, and Nate—thank you for building my beautiful garden and fence when I wasn't strong enough to do it myself. It's that same garden I've looked at through my window everyday while writing this book.

Special thanks to Amie for your relentless IIN talk and food and garden wisdom.

Thank you to Joshua, the Integrative Nutrition team and all IINers who continue to make ripples and waves—I am grateful to be a part of that inspiring community.

My appreciation to Dr. Hedlund and my cancer team at MCCM. And to my incredible surgeon, Dr. Donegan: Thank you for your skill, assertiveness and for bringing the luck o' the Irish!

And last, but not least: To my amazing co-author, Annette, my thanks to you for going on this adventure with me and for bringing along creativity, patience, motivation, diligence, humor, organization and your vocabulary shower curtain.

Index

Subject Index

A

Acupuncture, 37–38

Adrenal-support foods, 156–158

Agricultural practices, 117–118

Alternative medicine, 35–36

Animal foods, reducing, 11

Animal protein, 10–11, 78, 91–93, 96, 115–116, 135, 155

Anticancer: A New Way of Life, 82

Antioxidants, 68, 73–77, 82, 92, 151–153, 180

Anxiety, 21, 30, 32, 144, 187

Artificial sweeteners, 82–83, 113–115

B

Bach Flower tinctures, 184

Beans, 78–79, 256–267. **See also** Recipe Index

Berkey, Catherine, 90

Berries, 70–71

Beverages, 73–74, 116–117, 308–318. **See also** Recipe Index

Blood-healthy foods, 148–150

Body, and food, 22–27, 39–42, 107–108, 148–171, 187

Body, signs from, 104–106

Bone density, 66

Brain-healthy foods, 150–151

Breakfasts, 66, 102–103, 110, 121, 130–132, 157, 206–216. **See also** Recipe Index

Breathing exercises, 32

C

Cacao, 180

Cancer
causes of, 6–7
diagnosis of, 12, 16, 20, 24–25, 43–44
as full-time job, 28–31
life after, 188
preventing, 9–10
second opinions on, 29–30

Cancer survivors, 11–12

Cancer World, 16–17

Cancer-food link, 39–42, 107–108

Care Pages, 34

Caring Bridge, 34

Carotenoid-rich vegetables, 68, 76

Cheese, 88–90

"Chemo brain," 150

Chemotherapy treatments, 12, 21–22, 26–27, 140–143, 169–171

Chewing tips, 142

Children and change, 124–127

Chocolate, 172, 180–181

Coconut water, 117, 122, 161–162

Comfort foods, 165–168

Complementary medicine, 35–36

Constipation remedies, 159–161

Conventional medicine, 34–35

Cooking equipment, 119–120, 192–193

Cooking fun, 109

Cooking tips, 118–120

Cravings, 138–140

Creativity, 154

Cruciferous vegetables, 67–68, 76. **See also** Vegetables

Cultured foods, 75–76, 79–80, 115–116

D

Dairy foods, 88–90

Dancing, 108, 109, 186

Dark chocolate, 172, 180–181

Decision-making issues, 31–34

Depression, 87, 145, 175, 181

Desserts, 80, 132, 296–307. **See also** Recipe Index

Detoxifying foods, 151–153, 158. **See also** Antioxidants

Diet
changes in, 11, 22–27
changing in steps, 92–93, 99–101, 110–112, 121
recommendations for, 10–11
whole foods diet, 95–111

Dining out, 134–135

Recipe Index